The Normal Diet

DR. GLENN A. CLEARIE

ISBN 979-8-88751-495-6 (paperback)
ISBN 979-8-88751-496-3 (digital)

Christian Faith Publishing
832 Park Avenue
Meadville, PA 16335
www.christianfaithpublishing.com

The information provided in this publication is for informational purposes only and is not intended as a substitute for professional medical advice, diagnosis, or treatment. Readers are advised to consult with a qualified healthcare professional before making any health changes. No information in this book should be used to diagnose, treat, or cure any disease condition.

Printed in the United States of America

CONTENTS

INTRODUCTION

At first glance, you may have wondered, "What exactly is *The Normal Diet*, and why do we need some so-called and self-proclaimed expert telling me what is *normal* for me?" What you should be thinking is, why do we even need someone telling us how or what or when to eat in the first place? To this I would agree! It is from that perspective that I found the motivation to put pen to paper.

Nevertheless, the current health status of our country generally and our communities specifically is degrading before our very eyes. So we need…something more. My prayer is that this is a part of that *something more.*

After countless years, countless books, and countless health professionals in all nutritional advisory and counseling capacities, we find ourselves sicker, fatter, and more drugged than at any other time in our history.

Dare I even begin to say that it may very well be because of all the experts that we find ourselves in this challenging place to begin with. Science, politics, and corporate entities have had its fun while ruining our health; now it's time to turn them off altogether. If being uninformed gets you healthier, then get uninformed!

So how can another "diet" book even come close to making a difference? I surmise it's because it's not a diet book but, in fact, quite the opposite. More of an anti-diet book.

Yes, of course, we will be speaking about food and dietary consumption. However, so much more is involved, and some of it isn't pleasant in the short term.

Think of the ensuing topics and material we will cover as more of a candid talk among friends rather than the business-as-usual dos and don'ts flow chart that once you diverge from you consider yourself a failure. All bestselling diet programs are typically short-lived among the masses. *The Normal Diet*, however, is based upon a sustenance approach that has kept us alive for thousands of years. Now that's what I call a track record!

So many diets, more specifically fad diets, are generally exclusionary in nature. Most look to limit or exclude your intake of one of the macro nutrients, protein, carbohydrates, or fats. *The Normal Diet* wants you to include all three abundantly. *Abundantly* doesn't mean overconsumption; it means with a joyous spirit, knowing that what you are eating is feeding your body and fueling you in the correct way, not tearing you down and helping disease to fester.

Perhaps the biggest offender of imposing an exclusionary fad type diet is our own government criteria vis-à-vis our national food pyramid. Sure, that's working out well, isn't it?

Here is another thing about exclusionary fad type diets. While they tend to lead to singling out one or more of the macronutrients—fat, carbohydrates, or protein they can also overshoot the target by recommending their perceived must have micronutrients, i.e., minerals and vitamins like calcium. Enough about calcium already! Hence, we end up with "do this, don't eat that" and the "take this and don't take that" mentality that has led to an enriched and engineered food society and RDA (recommended daily allowance) following zombies. Foolishness.

Isn't it logical to eat the Normal Diet that we were meant to eat and let our bodies handle the assimilation of what it needs? We have over thought the most basic of survival instincts—nourishment. We now find ourselves in a society that believes we need others to tell us how to fend for ourselves. We are led to believe we just couldn't do it without the experts. How embarrassing for us that we have bought into such nonsense intellectually, emotionally, and monetarily!

The good news to all is that we can each decide our own path to follow. We ourselves, working within the framework of all things legal can make our own choices. The choice to move from a place of sickness to the place of better health is an individual choice, your choice. Not the governments, not your medical doctor, not your shrinks, or anyone else for that matter. You alone are responsible for you. When it comes to the *diseases of lifestyle* that make up the vast majority of illness, you need to come to grips that it is *your fault* whether you are sick or healthy. Of course, exception to this blanket statement exists, yet taking sole responsibility for your past, current, and future health takes all the nonsense out of the equation. You are responsible for you. End of story.

This premise of "it is your responsibility" is paramount to *The Normal Diet* lifestyle. No crybabies. No feeling sorry for yourself. Just acceptance pure and simple. It's freeing in a way, isn't it? Don't get stressed about having to take responsibility for another thing. We are going to take it slow and march ahead. If we need to drag you a little before you can crawl and then walk, well, okay, so be it.

Since you're choosing to read this book, then I must assume that you want to be healthier because if you wanted to get sicker, you wouldn't need a book. You could just keep listening to the ads on the radio, in the magazines, on television, overhead billboards, and easily achieve sickness in no time! Most have chosen this path. Just look around you. Maybe look in the mirror.

The bad news to doing something about your health status is that, like me, you may become an outcast in your own village. Okay, that's a bit extreme, but if you need to, want to, and decide to change or implement what needs to be done, you had better accept the scrutiny, ridicule, and discouragement that goes along with it.

The wall you come up against isn't always going to be your mother-in-law! That was a joke. The resistance may be your spouse, children, friends, your doctor, or employer. No easy answer to who will try to knock you down, but just be aware that it occurs frequently.

For sure, big pharma and industrial food and beverage creators do not want you to succeed in this regard. They want you and your whole family on their drugs and franken-food as much as I want you on broccoli!

Come to understand that "for every idea, there is an equal and opposite criticism." So get used to the idea of roadblocks coming your way and decide to move on and succeed anyway. The saving grace is that once you achieve your objectives, the dissident few will either fade away or slap you on the back and say, "I knew you could do it." Yeah, thanks.

Based on my experience in this regard, I suggest keeping quiet about anything and everything you are doing until the positive changes are so evident that people are commenting and asking questions.

Now maybe you are thinking that what is normal to one person isn't normal to another. When you take into account the different cultural or religious culinary lifestyles you could make a case for this viewpoint. However, the Normal Diet is more concerned about the debacle of the western diet that has diluted and quite candidly wiped out the majority of culinary eloquences that existed in our country just a generation ago.

Our great-grandparents, in most cases now, our grandparents, wouldn't know the first thing about shopping in a modern-day grocery store. They would just keep wondering where all the groceries were and where the food was hiding!

I can imagine my Scottish granny expressing her astonishment at all the pseudo-food. Sure, the produce aisle may be easier for her or anyone of us to navigate, but the rest of the store would sure lead to a puzzled look, confusion, disbelief, and then dismay at how far, not in a good way, we have come. My guess is she would pick out a box of tea and leave.

Much of present-day supermarket foods resemble food or imitates the shape of food in some fashion but isn't. Much like going to a wax museum where wax people look like the real person, most of what we consume has replaced legitimate food.

Perhaps *The Normal Diet* caught your eye because you are in fact one of those individuals who follows fad programs looking for the quick and easy way to get skinny, fit a bathing suit, or attend your thirty-year high school reunion. Again, this isn't that type of book.

Does this mean that this should be the end-all-tell-all omnivores guide to the eating galaxy? Geez, I sure hope not. If all you ever do is listen to me, you are in trouble for sure! You need to start listening to your own body and that's what I am here to help you do.

I can tell you that the Normal Diet is the correct way that 99 percent of us should approach the foods and liquids and all other edible items of sorts that exist in all of creation.

Now, how is that for an introduction.

Essential Understanding

All of us should have a common health goal: that being to remain healthy for as long as we are able and then die quickly with our dignity intact at a ripe older age. This is a worthy goal to aspire too. To this end, let us give attention to some basic thoughts/paradigms and principles that we need to consider in order to reach our full health potential.

Keep an open mind. Do not shut off at the first sign of something you disagree with. Just keep an open mind and simply…consider. For sure, there will be many contemplations. Always is and should be. Take time to allow these new perspectives and thoughts to be ruminated on. Why wouldn't you? Work to understand how any suggestion, idea, concept, or recommendation could impact your health status. Allow yourself to see what you are willing to do at this moment in time. Just don't shut down completely.

Understand where you came from. Largely, our upbringing plays a large role in who we are and what we consume. In all cases? Maybe not, but most often, we are the products of our upbringing. Dietary consumption is not immune to it. So be ready to recognize the differences between what you do because of indoctrination, like drinking Fresca because your grandmother did (true story here, my grandmother loved Fresca and bought it for us when we were young. Tea was her absolute favorite, however, as it is now mine!) and eating dessert every night because "that's what you do and always have" versus what you should be doing given your particular bodily needs.

Forgive and move on. I would also ask that you forgive yourself for past mistakes, failures, and any future blunders that you may have made or in fact *will* make. Don't be so hard on yourself anymore. Maybe this is your first pass-through, or maybe you have tried many times before with not a stitch of success or improved health to show for it. Maybe you feel worse in some fashion. To this I would say that it's okay and that the reason it is taking so long is that you still have something to learn. I know that I do for sure. Once the lesson is learned, you are usually able to move forward.

Now as far as the Normal Diet goes, yes, we will of course cover *diet* parameters as clearly this is a primary reason you are reading this now. That said, being fully cognizant of *why* your health is important to you is paramount to finally making the changes you desire and having lasting long-term success. I want this book to help you achieve a renewal of your mind as much as your body. Because I do, we will veer into conversations that at the outset appear to be as far from nutrition as one could get. Know that these discussions will have a dramatic impact on your reasoning and perspective and bring much into focus that may have fallen to the wayside.

It is time for you to become centered again.

Would you agree that for the most part, we all have some degree of understanding of what we should and shouldn't be doing when it comes to our nutrition and health? I think you do. However, for some reason, the fruit turns moldy on the counter, and our salad mixes go bad in the fridge, yet all the chips, cookies, cakes, and favored snacks magically disappear…into our mouths.

So stay with me cover to cover. This won't take too long. In fact, *The Normal Diet* is intentionally condensed so that you can make clear-minded headway in a timely fashion. My hope is that somehow and in some way, you will come into your own essential understanding of who you are and why you do what you do, and are finally ready to get really healthy again. Once the shift occurs, there is no going back!

Now let's get going.

1

The Normal Diet Quick Start

I t is human nature to shoot first and point later. This approach typically leads to mistakes and *annoyingly* needing to circle back to the beginning and start again. However, it is common. I know for myself that once I decide on something, I want to have forward momentum as timely as possible. Once I make a decision, I just get after it, right or wrong; that is who I am.

As an example, when I get a new electronic device or need to assemble something, I look to see if a brief summary or quick start set of instructions are available. Just tell me what I gotta do, and I will get going and figure out the landscape as it presents itself.

Are you this way? Most people are. I shouldn't say *most*, I should say *many*. If they weren't, they wouldn't generally have quick start instructions as is so common across all categories.

I personally want to cut to the chase when able. This approach has enabled me to get a lot done and has led to success in many areas of my life. As you might imagine, this has also led to circling back to the beginning to correct the mistakes I have made by getting ahead of myself. Well, okay, let's chalk this up to human nature.

Ever so, why wouldn't we dedicate some discussion to how you could move the needle forward on your own behalf as it relates to bodily nutrition and health before even finishing this page. You can make course corrections down the road, but for the time being, let's make some decisions together that provide you a path and an understanding of sorts. Don't make me say a journey of a thousand miles begins with the first step.

The Normal Diet quick start should not detract from the overall premise that the diet isn't a diet but a *way of life* that we should have been normally traversing our whole lives!

That said, in the beginning, there are some actionable items that should be considered so you can hit the ground running. I want to make the transition as easy as possible, so here we go:

1. Clean your fridge and pantry. It feels *so good* to get a fresh start, and this is part of it. Throw out all needless snacks, cookies, and/or treats. Toss out anything and everything you know in your heart just should not be in the house.
2. Create an area or shelf that you can keep all your supplements, powders, herbals close at hand.
3. Purchase a blender. I prefer the magic bullet. If you like juicing as I do, then order a quality juicing machine. I currently have a Breville, and it is fantastic. Worth its weight in gold as far as I am concerned.
4. Check your weight. You may not want to but do it anyway. Simply observe where you are at with no feelings either way.
5. Check your blood sugars. I have utilized a simple store-bought glucometer for many years, and it really is amazing how this awareness helps overall.
6. Purchase containers that are BPA-free. A couple for water. A couple for smoothies on the go.
7. Pick five vegetables, three fruits, and two protein sources that you would enjoy over the next seven to ten days, purchase them, and of course eat them. Repeat.
8. Consider which whole food protein-based smoothie powder most agrees with you and get some. For decades, I have been using Standard Process *Complete*. They now have chocolate and vanilla as well as dairy-free.

9. Start gently stretching your body for a couple minutes in the morning and night. Maybe five minutes each time.
10. Purchase some light weights. Nothing fancy nor expensive. Start with dumbbells that you can use for many exercises; 10 lb., 15 lb., 20 lb., or thereabouts depending. If you need a 5 lbs or less, then get one. You be the judge.

These quick-start actionable steps are sound advice in advance preparation for what we are about to talk about. Of course, individuality comes into play, and we could add or take away from the above if we knew the exact situation presenting. However, we do not so take it for what it is.

I can share that while you implement, change, alter your nutrition and health lifestyle you should anticipate *suffering* a bit. That's something you do not want to hear, but it is true more often than not. Know that various bumps in the road can and may or will occur. Deal with it…or you will have to potentially deal with something worse later on.

Nobody can predict what will happen when you stop treating your body like a human landfill and start cleaning up the terrain. You could become constipated or have diarrhea. Maybe you have great energy or significant fatigue. Could a skin rash occur? Who knows… but *you* will once we get going!

Look, if you stopped drinking coffee, would you get a massive headache? Most would; I have, and it is not pleasant. However, that's not a good rationale to keep drinking a pot a day. At some point, we all pay the piper. The pain of discipline or the pain of regret you ultimately decide. When you pay the price or how steep it is, is on you. Always has been.

If you change nothing, nothing will change. You are about to change something, and something *will* change. I hope it's all good from start to finish yet let's go into this with both eyes open. You didn't "get this way overnight," so prepare as best you can and respond as best you can to what occurs.

Going slow is far more beneficial then going ballistic right from the start. Take it easy on yourself. I understand you want change *now*.

You want benefit *now*. Don't worry next year will be *"now"* before you know it!

Take to heart the quick-start considerations yet settle it in your mind that you are now playing the long game. This should immediately calm you down. We have no need for haste. Now let's go back to the start and *absorb and digest* what *The Normal Diet* is all about.

2

It's Personal

Don't be charmed or fooled. Your health is and always will be as personal as it gets. Don't make a mistake in letting your health become defined by any person, program, diet, product, prescription, group, or organization. This includes spouses, friends, family, doctor, anyone, or anything that attempts to capture and contain your growth and progress, including your emotional self, which so often sabotages the best of intentions.

I guess this is the part where I should counter my statements and say that there are agencies, programs, et cetera that can make a difference. However, we need a fresh perspective, a generational type of perspective that goes far beyond our weekly "weigh-ins" and daily "points."

When I say that it is personal doesn't mean secretive or solo. Just keep it personal. As in, "This is who I am and what I do (or now I do), and it is not for debate anymore."

I have been in the practice of health and healing for more than twenty-five years and counting. I have been witness to much baloney in the health improvement category. I can say with some relative authority that by and large much of what has always been effective is a "steady as she goes" approach and has very little to do with some doctor or health care professional telling you what to do. You need to start thinking for yourself again and reclaim the *lost art of common sense*. The information that keeps coming at us is just noise, distractions in fact from our main purpose, that being improved natural health.

Have you ever looked to see just how much research on health and nutrition is being pumped out on a regular basis? Or how about the plethora of books, magazines, and other media platforms that spew nutrition information at nauseam. Are we better off for it? I don't think we are.

Clearly, research on the topic is important; nobody would disagree. However, it is as if once something new is discovered, a profit center is not too far behind. Interestingly, though, it appears that if there is no anticipated profit at the end of the research, then there just isn't research done to begin with. In all cases? Of course not yet; see this for the truth this is. Do you really need scientific experimenters to tell you what's in an apple before you will eat it? Does an apple need to have full disclosure of its constituents before it can do you good once eaten? That's crazy talk. Just eat the apple already; nowadays, it's probably four a day…

Research has revealed to us that antioxidants could potentially help to stabilize free radicals, thereby assisting our human bodies in perhaps numerous ways such as slow the aging process; help those with type-2 diabetes, cancers, cardiovascular disease, and neurodegenerative conditions. Are we better off knowing this? At the outset, we must say yes, just like having landed on the moon is progress so is uncovering and identifying *things* that have the potential to improve life.

That said, understand that all research draw conclusions. It is supposed to, right? Is it too early to be bold enough to state that the research performed and subsequent conclusion(s) can oftentimes be left up to interpretation and/or "artistic license"? Don't make me say *manipulated* as I am doing my best to not be cynical nor sound like a conspiracy theorist. I am simply calling it like I see it. As in the antioxidant example, the product push, based upon the research has become vast and extremely profitable. Vitamins A, C, and E are antioxidants in their own right and popular overall. So it is not surprising to see their *research-based* inclusion in so many products we use day in and day out. I am not saying this is bad or otherwise. However, it is commonplace. Whether hair products, oral supplements, liquids or facial and/or body cremes, you could find that the supporting antioxidant validity is a basis if not *the* basis for the marketing campaign(s).

If you didn't know, there is another opinion and viewpoint about the antioxidants example that we could put forth as validated by research. As crazy as it sounds, it is also recognized that free radicals *may not* always be that bad and actually assist with cell division *and* could or do help cells talk to each other. So let's not throw out the baby with the bathwater here. I feel we are pretty certain that too many free radicals hanging around can spin into something not so good for our human bodies. It seems appropriate to conclude this; however, I wonder if this position will be seen as archaic in another fifty years.

So yes, antioxidant supplements like vitamin C, vitamin E, and vitamin A may help in *many* ways…or perhaps just in *some* ways or *at least* can't hurt you or maybe should not hurt you—actually, who really knows anyway.

Let's just say that the basic communication is that antioxidants are good and free radicals bad; now buy the product.

But truly, are we, have we been better off now knowing this information? If we say yes, then should everyone be on these supplements daily? What about all the other researched products that conclude or almost conclude that if you take *that*, you will enjoy benefit X and/or outcome Z.

A more reasonable approach would be simply to consume broccoli, spinach, carrots, and potatoes and all the rest that are all high in antioxidants. Avocados is another. So many more high-antioxidant value food sources exist and, in my humble opinion, may have a greater impact on overall health than a singled-out lab-produced pill.

Now perhaps you are thinking that a blend of supplements and actual food may be the best approach, and I do feel that approach has credence and could be discussed further.

That said, getting back to our discoveries, is life expectancy or health status any better knowing what nutritional research has uncovered? Yes, the research is necessary, but again, it can give mixed messages and lead to confusion. One day, research validates a certain vitamin then the next it refutes its benefit. What is the public to do?

Inevitably, through the trickle-down effect, this research-validated information gets communicated to the end user, that being you and me. Maybe this information is shared in a consultation-type meeting with your doctor or nutritionist. Maybe it was from an ad in the paper or infomercial on TV selling a product.

For example, let's consider that this information is about the superior antioxidant known as resveratrol.

Resveratrol is a naturally occurring polyphenol that resides within a host of plant species. You may already know that it is found in the skin of grapes; hence when you think of wine, particularly red wine, we tend to think that it's the resveratrol content that could benefit us.

Now that may be very well true, and I think it is to some degree. But is alcohol generally really that good for you? No, it isn't. We still drink it anyway, though, don't we?

At any rate, resveratrol may have antibacterial, antiviral, and antifungal benefits. It may also arguably have antioxidant benefits. When you have a high resveratrol level in dry red wine, it will actually help you to dance easier, yet that, of course, after a bottle or two…

My guess is that if a company sells a resveratrol supplement, and they do, or resveratrol food like products such as drinks, cremes, and oral supplementation, then they would market and promote their wares heavily based on the research findings.

This is another example and reminder that a business wants and needs to sell something. That's what they do. Hot dog stands sell hot dogs, pizza places sell pizza, and on and on. I sell health. So it is no different in our imaginary case where the resveratrol makers want to sell resveratrol products. Given validated research, they are empowered to sell with zeal.

What I want you to consider is that perhaps at some point in the future, "other" research could refute or minimize resveratrol's claims. Now I am not getting down on resveratrol; in fact, I think it is a powerhouse nutrient. I am attempting to stress that regaining and maintaining your health is absolutely, positively personal and intimate. Its huge! There is no aspect to our vitality that isn't personal, so don't treat yourself flippantly anymore. So whichever you invest your time, talents, and treasure in better be worth it. That said, your health is a treasure so spend wisely here.

So yes, you probably could benefit from resveratrol or many other research validated micronutrients, but I am pretty sure that the unadulterated whole food concept such as grapes, blueberries, pistachios that inherently have resveratrol residing within, is a better approach and leads to better outcomes than others combined. Why, might you ask? Well, my answer would simply be "Because God ordained the plan since before the beginning of time." How's that for a boast!

Stop thinking impersonally about your health. The Bible says that lukewarm water should be spit out of the mouth! Meaning, take a stance. Be hot or cold, but don't think about your health so laissez-faire anymore!

Whenever I see a social media post about the next new supplement I am missing out on, I chuckle. Usually behind the curtain, you find more of the same no matter which professional is pushing their wares. Clearly, the Normal Diet endorses the use of appropriate supplements. More than not, however, we need to consider whole food-based supplements, not synthetic. We will touch on this soon, yet for now, know there is a significant difference and together we will explore that genre.

The point of this is to draw attention that you are the professional here. Your innate intelligence that dwells inside takes care of countless operational functions. It is actually quite staggering when you take a moment to think about it! All we really need to do is provide proper sustenance, and boom, we are off to the races.

Look, the Normal Diet is simple. In fact, your ever-functioning innate that *transcends your conscious ability to control or direct*—think, heart beating or intestinal digestion, is taking care of *everything* as we speak to a significant degree. So all you really need to do is help it along a little with nutrients to keep the furnace burning, and your body will take care of the rest. What we are to discuss will do just that! While I assert that the Normal Diet is simple, it isn't easy. The reason for this is threefold:

- Many make the mistake thinking a gimmick, supplement, or piece of exercise equipment is going to come along and take care of everything for you. It isn't.
- Ingrained lifelong patterns have built certain ways of thinking, eating, acting, being that are on autopilot. Time to retool all that!
- You lack *consistency* in your approach to address your health.

We don't live in a bubble. We live in the real world where we are inundated with "stuff." The media rams this *stuff* down our psyches with such hype and repetition that we become numb to and then generally accept the *stuff* as, for a lack of better term, valid.

Case in point, the complete acceptance of our society, specifically our children that medicine is what we do to keep us healthy and treat conditions. Aren't our kids indoctrinated from a very young age that virtually every condition can be addressed with a pill? Every second or third commercial tells them so, and it becomes embedded. What a great marketing ploy that the indoctrination to pill popping starts way back in our youth when we are told to pop medicinal gummies.

Could you even imagine the positive impact if every second or third commercial was about fruits and vegetables keeping you healthy, strong, and its ability to correct most illnesses? Imagine that well-intentioned and appropriately directed indoctrination! Would be a game changer from my natural perspective.

At any rate, we as adults are inundated by similar "stuff." How many times have you seen infomercials that have an authority figure being interviewed one on one and endorse the products they are selling? My guess is you have seen this repeatedly over the years. If the equipment, product, and service is good enough for our favorite celebrities, then by golly, it must be good for me too!

I myself have indeed purchased items over the years that were endorsed by celebrities. Admittedly, I do have the Total Gym, and it is a great piece of equipment. I also have a nautilus and free weights and pull-up bar and a bunch of other stuff my family and I use. Some more than others.

However, it is the realization that these pieces of equipment, these products aren't doing the work or making the changes. You are. Look, a gym membership doesn't do anyone any good unless you act. The only one who profits from it is the gym owner.

Always the introspective individual, I guess the same could be said of this book. Without action, the only one who profits is myself from the sale of my book(s). Do you know how many times I have thought and/or said that "whoever invented that sport, activity, piece of equipment really wanted chiropractors to do well!" Case in point could be the sport of cheerleading. I am convinced that wrestling was also created so the chiropractic profession would always be gainfully employed.

You really need to take some time, sit quietly, and truly give thought to whether or not you believe that your God-given beautiful body can simply do its job without product X, service Y, or person Z.

The second point to consider is whether your belief system is or is not in alignment with the actions you are taking or advised to take. "Something" that is not aligned as it should be causes stress, strife, and sickness. From what I have witnessed, there is simply a lack of congruency within oneself that strikes to the heart of the matter more often than not. It's as if we are each double-minded. This awful situation has ruined more than health—it has ruined marriages, relationships, and all the rest that humans can be involved with. Acknowledgment of such and then identification is critical at the outset. You can lie to others; just stop lying to yourself already.

If you have not yet evaluated yourself on the deepest inner levels, faced the *imposter syndrome* within, or ripped the scab off the truth of your nature, whatever that may be, then we shouldn't start marching forward. It will be and usually lead to disaster, failure, or discouragement. You need to "drink the Kool-Aid" as they say. Jump in with both feet. Burn the ships you came to the island on so that you can never go back the same way.

With that said, let's also just stop blaming mommy, daddy, a boss, or whomever else. Enough already. Grow up and take stock of self. We are adults here. This is a serious discussion about how you will be living out the *rest* of your life. I say you live well and healthy.

In his book, *The 7 Habits of Highly Effective People*, Mr. Stephen Covey coins the term "inside out" which he defines as "starting first with self," your character, your principles, your motives, then and only then is it worthwhile to take the next step.

He elaborates,

> The inside-out approach says that private victories precede public victories, that making and keeping promises to ourselves precedes making and keeping promises to others. It is futile to put personality ahead of character, to try to improve relationships with others before improving ourselves.

I couldn't agree more!

Commitment, congruency, consistency is key to better outcomes in all of life's categories.

If we keep this front and center in our lives, can you even imagine how amazing your future will be? All I ask of you presently is to apply this in relation to the food you ingest.

Along the same lines of reasoning, I recently was discussing with my daughters the importance of goals being aligned with their core standards. As a father, one would hope my wife and I instilled good values and above-board standards into each of their psyches. Since I believe this to be true, the natural expectation is that their life's path reflects their solid footing.

I would hope that after all these years, they don't have a goal to rob a bank. That would be absurd. That's not even a consideration—how could it be? That's about as far from aligned with who they as a person can get. I also anticipate that their diets will generally be filled with wholesome nourishment more often than not. In addition, I naturally expect that as they continue to mature through their life cycle, they will consistently perform appropriate exercise, stretching, and strength training. I know they will. Why? Because first and foremost, they have it settled on the inside. I hope this illustration gets the point across, that being, much of the Normal Diet is predicated on truth with oneself on many levels.

In our approach, we need to think clearly, and this is clearly the approach we need to take.

Again, *this is personal!* Without working on the innermost recesses of yourself, you will end up where you may have always found yourself—failing and giving up.

It doesn't have to be that way.

For some, that long hard look to the inside yields an emotional issue that's raging like a lion, looking to devour anything in its path. For others, it might be a physical trait, characteristic, gene, or trauma-induced condition that you feel is a handicap of sorts. Face yourself, your fears, your doubts *now* in any way that is appropriate and let's get it over with and move on.

Are we talking about quitting smoking or drinking? Maybe. Could it be getting involved with a support group, ending a destructive relationship or work environment? It varies significantly from one to the next, but I am quite certain that each of us have one or two issues that need to be resolved on the inside. It will do wonders for you to resolve and confront whatever it is that has been undermining your health goals.

The greatest battles don't exist in the physical; they exist in our minds!

So take this personally or don't even bother to read on.

Now of the three, consistency is what I see as the single biggest derailment to the best of intentions. Everyone is good out of the gate. It's when the pain kicks in that the pack begins to pull away and leaves us behind with mud on our face.

Consistency is the glue that pulls everything else together. Inherent to consistency is a time component that cannot be separated from it. Consistent for an hour may be where you start yet as you lean into the new you, the time component of consistency will, naturally, as it needs to be, become increasingly longer and longer. The result of which will lead to not just a new habit or new lifestyle or reap of the reward—it leads to a new person on the inside. Who doesn't desire for personal growth in this way!

To the point, transition from where you are to where you want to move toward involves a few moving parts yet to truly be determined. Again, an important aspect is to spend time with yourself in introspection and self-understanding. It takes evaluation of certain key things about yourself or at the very least recognizing certain traits, aspects, habits, shortcomings, etc., and yes, this takes some time. The long and short of it all is that clearly your health is a deeply personal matter. Remember this as you move along.

3

Grassroots Effort

Now all individuals, including our health care professionals themselves, can and do have health issues. Your doctors, dieticians, nutritionist, therapist, etc., are not immune from whatever you yourself may find yourself facing. Obesity, trauma, anxiety, autoimmune, and all the rest obviously are fair game as since we are all human then we all be can surely be afflicted by all things human.

Perhaps what I am getting at here is that if you are looking for the perfect guru to guide you all way to whatever goal you are looking for then allow me to say you will be waiting a long time. Better to be following a limping general than a straight-backed lieutenant.

This is true in all things, isn't it? I laugh when I see politicians who hold themselves out as above reproach. It's usually those that do that are truly downright diabolical and on the take. Same with our faith leaders. How many have fallen from grace? In fact, any and all have the ability to be depraved, and we know that anyone can fall prey at any time. I do not suppose to be above the pail. I am aware that I can have a major face plant at any time. Regarding the Normal Diet, you may one day see me chowing down a whole pizza with one hand and chocolate cheesecake with the other. You never know!

With this said, you do not necessarily need to discount the counsel given from said individual. Yes, they, me, we may be hypocritical, yet the message delivered could be spot on. Should your morbidly obese and diabetic medical doctor be telling you to avoid sugar you should listen instead of judging. Am I right? I think I am. Take good counsel regardless of the source.

"I find myself doing what I don't want to do and not doing what I truly desire to do" (Romans 7:15–20). Such a bold assertion by the apostle Paul surmises that state of us humans, doesn't it? His position taken and discussed strikes deep. Such a statement allows for the continuing realization that we are all fully human and, well, flawed. Nonperfect, if you will. No one escapes this category unless, possibly, you are a robot. Please check to see if you have a belly button. If you do, then you fall into the first category of the nonperfect and should feel right at home with the rest of us.

Knowing and accepting the nature of who we are and our shortcomings, allows for, or should allow for, a sense of calm, knowing that each and every human that has walked or will walk on the ground beneath our feet has flaws and royally screwed up at one point or another. It gives me a sense of freedom in preparing this much-needed and timely viewpoint on the sad situation that exists in the imperfections in the "nutritional realm" and its impact on our country and world at large.

Striving to better ourselves is what we imperfect creatures aspire to or should aspire to. The purpose of life is to have a life of purpose. Mine is to help others live enriched lives through better health. However, compared to some, I am less healthy than they are. Can I match physique with an Arnold Schwarzenegger? No, of course not. It's not how we compare to others it is more about where we are at and where we are going in our personal journey. It's about you in comparison to the *you*, you want to and can become.

So without reservation, I'll confess that I fall short of the optimum state of health that I would wish for myself. A similar confession from you in the beginning is also required for us all to drop our guards and move on without pride or prejudice. The epiphany and humbling nature of it all is in realizing this and moving forward in faith, hope, and expectancy of better days and better health ahead.

The liberties that I must take are from a viewpoint of an individual who represents the ever-elusive epitome of superior health. This is a state not achieved by anyone but is striven for by many. A worthy crusade. A worthy goal.

To that end, I cannot with a clear conscious cast the first stone at you without at least admitting that I should be dropping a boulder on myself. My shortcomings, my weaknesses, my mistakes are ever before me. In the nutritional context, I have had sugar once or twice. As a child, I have begged my mother for fast food on more than one occasion, and as an adult, I have been known to steal candy from children.

Heck, I even met my wife in Burger King! It was a first job for the both of us as kids. I cannot say that either of us have had anything from that fast-food chain in perhaps a decade or longer, yet I wouldn't put it past me! If I did, I would probably get a Double Whopper with Cheese, and then come back into the practice and tell people not to eat any of that garbage (laughing emoji face here).

Even though I drink plain teas daily and often, to this day, I still look forward to a cup of coffee, especially just after a long run. I still can hardly pass on the red-colored Twizzlers that my mother gave me sparingly as a kid. These days, I refer to this delightful plastic-like, diabetes-enhancing substance as *vitamin T*, somehow calling it that minimizes my guilt. So does it disqualify me for offering the solution to the risen tide of sickness? No. I perceive it validates.

I have had my fair share of adult beverages to the point of intoxication. One day, I decided I just didn't want that stuff in my body at all, and for the next seven years, I didn't. So I know a thing or two about self-indulgence and self-discipline, having experienced and continuing to experience them both. Just like you if I may be so bold.

So who better to write about a war than from someone who has been and is routinely on the front line? Clearly, the experience with food and nutrient intake pales in comparison to a military war, but this is a war on a different front nevertheless…and we are losing big time.

This "war," if you will, begins ultimately in the home, your home and with your mouth. It is your *grass root efforts* that can turn the tide and win the skirmishes and ultimately the battle for health, vitality, and longevity. Your health, the health of your children, grandchildren, and generations to come is at stake.

Should my tone be rather harsh, that's my intent. It needs to be at the outset. This is the real world here. Not an infomercial.

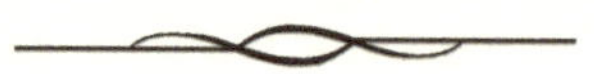

Only read on if, in fact, you are at a point where you yourself are ready to accept the "humanness" of yourself and others. Read on with the realization that what appears to be not always is. Smoke and mirrors, liposuction, gastric bypass, air brushing, advertising tactics, synthetic vitamins, and of course, prescription medicines are increasingly utilized with reckless abandon for more than the presumed goal of improving the health of our families. Sickness is big business. Please do not allow yourself to forget that.

Throughout my travels as a natural healthcare provider, I have of course come to have a certain perspective on things. What I have found is that not many want to hear it even though they are in fact paying me to hear it. It's almost as if the majority want to just have someone to validate what they are already doing even if it's absurd. "That's great, Tom, keep taking all eight prescriptions, you'll be fine."

If I stated what I felt on many situations without tempering, I wouldn't have but a handful of patients. Even family and friends for that matter. I learned from the great country singer Kenny Rogers, now deceased, that you have to know when to hold 'em, know when to fold 'em, know when to walk away, and know when to run. Great advice.

I find that initially being in relationship with a person is more important than hammering them for what they may be doing wrong whether inadvertently or intentionally. I have come to understand that my patients specifically need to be in a meaningful relationship with me and understand where I am coming from before they would even consider taking professional advice. It's true. Much of who we are, where we are, is built on relationships and our own unique experiences culminated through the years. Said another way, we each look at things through different lenses. Perspective does matter.

Over the past many years of providing health and wellness care, I have discovered various ways in which optimum health can manifest forth in each one of us. To bring this information to its intended recipient, you must not alienate them. Being committed to assisting those individuals that truly want better health, vitality, and longevity, you must "relax" until you earn their trust.

To jump in on the first encounter and tell them how disgusting their diet is and that their untimely and eminent death is knocking is no way to achieve this goal. On the other hand, telling them that it will just take a few weeks to correct thirty years of breaking down the human vessel they live in isn't quite the best approach either. Again, you need to know when to hold 'em, and holding your tongue is the best place to start.

Conversely, some individuals, and this may describe you, need the plain and hard facts. At times, I have needed to be more direct, but that can only be done after establishing the heart-to-heart connection.

Sometimes, however, you have to know when to fold 'em. That is a polite way to say that a person isn't ready or truly willing to make those pattern changes. Maybe at some point in the future, that person will be ready and able to implement what it requires to achieve better health.

Maybe that person who is finally ready is *you* right now.

Wherever all this finds you, I want to be clear that you absolutely can begin to transition into *the new you* at this very moment. The fundamentals we will surely outline always act as the fallback position from which to regroup should you mess things up dietarily, and clearly, we can and will. However, do not forget there is a whole lot more to all things diet than nutrition.

Of course, the quality of food ingested is paramount, yet so is how much you consume in one sitting. How about timing? That's pretty important as well, so let's not overlook that. Also, what specific combination of foods work well together and what doesn't could be a whole other tidbit to dive into.

Let's not forget about all the personal care products that we use day in and day out. Your body is *eating* all that as well. Toxic shampoos, antiperspirants, soaps, creams, gels, perfumes, and all the rest are absorbed via the skin, and the body needs to try to handle all that in addition to, let's say, your double mocha latte and gluten sugar muffin the mouth took in for breakfast. So we need to realize much if we are going to improve health, aren't we?

If you consider the logical nature of what I just expressed, you see things could be, or better stated, should be, quite easy to address. However, when we factor in what our minds "trick" us into doing you see that yes, bigger picture views of the circumstances involved have much influence on your nutrition at every turn.

This is why I went to great lengths to paint a personal picture of my own life that demonstrates the desire and wherewithal to maintain my good health yet fully living as a person who clearly could be doing a little better. This is common not the exception. This is a major consideration we need to understand and accept as we discuss the Normal Diet.

I find the self-imposed guilt surrounding what *we want to do* versus *what actually occurs* to be quite staggering in those I have cared for. It stops people in their tracks.

Listen here, if you want to gain back momentum in your life, you are going to have to move beyond the self-deprecation and loathing. Isn't that just getting old at this point? Sure, it is. So free yourself and allow a new frame of reference of self-awareness and a well-balanced love for self to mature.

It will take time, yet when you are on the other side of something you didn't want to eat, drink, say or do, you don't have to hate yourself for days anymore. No, in fact, I want you to simply show *grace* to yourself as you do for others.

When I speak of grassroots efforts, I mean it in more than one way. Foundationally, a new mindset needs to be awoken in you. Essentially, this is the key to it all. However, let's not minimize that I truly do mean a grassroots effort, as in *green-based food.*

It should come as absolutely no surprise that consuming more plant-based food sources will heal many woes. Pick any trouble humans have and you can be pretty sure eating better will improve it. That isn't even for debate—never was.

It is simply human nature that the want for sugar, caffeine, recreational drugs, alcohol, and other detrimental things supersedes, albeit momentarily, the desire for good health. I am not joking here. There is something deep within us that craves what is not healthy for us. Very strange? Yes, it is, however, a truth nonetheless.

Inherent to all things *health*, you have to eventually conclude and acknowledge this simple tenant that "green stuff"—i.e., all food sources in the plant realm—is the fulcrum on which vibrancy capitulates. *This* is the *grassroots effort* that must be front and center in your life.

There is no way around this, so please put what you do or don't like aside. No pill, potion, or elixir can replace this natural law. No piece of gym equipment neither. The grassroot effort you need to wrap your mind around is the *effort* you put into *root* (vegetables) and grass (green plant stuff) nutrition.

For this to be easily assimilated, it is the mindful-willful-emotional *you* that needs to take full stock and handle the childish side of self once and for all.

The truth of what I just stated bears out time and time again. Contemplate what we have covered here in this chapter deeply. Come to grips with the truth it is. Don't run from it and try to prove it wrong. You cannot.

4

The Whole Water Thing

To sum it up, just drink water. But that would be too easy, wouldn't it? So I should probably make everyone feel better by confusing the situation and making it difficult to understand the simple art of filling a glass with a clear fluid of H_2O.

I could give you a guide, as in drink half your body weight, in corresponding ounces of course, every day. I could just say drink a gallon of water every day. Maybe add in or subtract if you drink caffeinated beverages like coffee. We could talk about the fluid content that is inherent to our food and balance it with daily totals.

I have discussed all these and more at one time or another. But just like hand grenades, as they say, just get close to the target!

Now what type of water? We have distilled, spring, flavored, vitamin-enhanced, carbonated, caffeinated, and sport waters of all shapes and sizes. The darling as of late appears to be PH-balanced, aka alkaline water—it's actually what I prefer, yet let's not muddy the water here. Yes, pun intended.

When I was visiting Scotland many years ago, I met a man who had struck an underground spring. He owned the land and owned the mineral rights as well. This meant he owned whatever was underground more or less. In his case, it was water.

This gentleman started bottling this water in a very Pierre-type way. These were beautiful blue, tinted, wine-shaped, corked bottles.

He had named his particular brand after arguably the most famous person in all the land, Robert Burns. Robert Burns was an eighteenth-century poet. His contribution to the literary field is perhaps unrivaled to this day. My dearly beloved granny would recite him regularly. Oh, how I wish that youth wasn't wasted on the young as it is only in my later decades of life that I can appreciate her espousing such sweetness in her native tongue!

While you may be unfamiliar with his poetry, you may know Mr. Burns's poem he wrote in the late 1700s and later set to melody titled "Auld Lang Syne," the staple song that we greet each new year with; that is his work.

At any rate, this gentleman coined his natural spring water after Mr. Burns. He called it *Burns-well springwater*. The water itself has a high mineral content, the way water should. Minerals assist with all physiological functions. You need macro nutrients like proteins, fats, and carbs; however, do not neglect micronutrients, of which, minerals of all types help us to thrive.

I am giving a heavy-handed critique when I state that while minerals are fantastic to seek out, perhaps his water wouldn't be so well received here in the States. Now that is just my observation based on two reasons: The first being the high-mineral content I mentioned does have a rather distinct taste and aftertaste that many of us may not be accustomed to. Perhaps not as smooth, if I could describe it that way. The other is the name. *Burns-well*. The name itself is a bit off-putting. If you didn't know better, maybe you would think that it actually burns your throat on the way down. Who wants something that *burns* very *well*. Not me.

Okay, I did side track a bit at the expense of a true gentleman with a fine product, but it seemed too easy to pass up. To this day, I have bottles of *burns-well* water, both spring and bubbly, on display at my house. When I look at them, I can still almost taste that powerful mineral water that resides inside. Clean water should be the foundation for health that you need to build upon. Mineral water clearly is a fantastic option, yet let's keep it all simple as, again, I remind you to please simply drink water.

Recently, I was discussing the need for fluid intake with a patient who suffered with leg cramps. She admittedly did not take in much more than a glass or two of unsweetened tea every day. Unsweetened tea is a good decision, but I made recommendations that she drink "more water." I specifically asked her to drink spring water for a while because of the mineral content.

To my surprise, she adamantly opposed my recommendations to drink the spring water because it came in plastic bottles. "Don't you know that the plastic bottles leech harmful substances?" she stated with authority. Maybe I could have told my patient to drink directly from a trickling spring, but what would she say about the pesticide run off from the farm?

It took me a moment and then I quietly responded, "Well, what about that diet soda you're drinking?"

It is not surprising that each and every single one of us have something we enjoy for whatever reason that is not healthy for ourselves, yet we do it anyway. You have things you do that clearly are not improving your health and I have mine. That said, just add water consumption to your life, and I can virtually guarantee that in some way, your life will improve. Is that a wide net? Yes, water is that important.

Truth be told, anywhere you turn, you can get varying advice of which water product is the best for you and the containers they do or don't come in. Ask enough people, and you will see endless opinions on the matter. All arguments seemingly have their merits until you become a person lost in the desert, at which point, you would not care one way or another as you would be begging for whatever was at the ready. Please simply drink water.

My uncle has told me since I was knee-high that water is *no good* for you. When I would ask him why, he would say, "Do you know what fish do in water?" He would then tell me to get him a scotch and hold the water. That joke never ever gets old because it's based in truth!

Perhaps consider installing a filtration system if you have concerns about contaminants, but the residential designs generally do not filter out the smallest of particles like fluoride. The reverse osmosis filters would, however.

A good idea would be to distill your own water like I did in my home for more than a decade. But doesn't that lead to demineralization of bone if followed long-term? I have heard that said on many occasions. When my then young daughter happened to break her wrist while innocently playing, I questioned whether this was the case. Our family does in fact take a wholefood multimineral supplement regularly since that time.

In *The Normal Diet*, you drink water more often than not. Period.

I will take a stance on the subject and say that I prefer alkaline water when able and have purchased a permanent system. These current systems are really not that expensive, and I do believe the benefit is worth it. As mentioned, I also have a home-based kettle-like pot that distills water. For so many years, I was making distilled water each day. It costs a few hundred dollars for the coffee pot-like distiller and replacement charcoal cartridges cost a few dollars every month or so. Now that I have my alkaline and purification system, I don't do this as much.

I do not like to drink distilled water from purchased bottles as I do not want to take a chance that scalding hot water, whether distilled or otherwise, is put into a plastic bottle. The high temperatures will add to the leeching of the chemicals from the bottle.

I feel I must give you my opinion and state that I am convinced that all the fluorinated and chlorinated water is just toxic to our bodies. I have read on the subject and that's my conclusion. However, while I have replaced all showerheads to filter out what we could I have showered in, washed my hands in, and swam in the very "contaminated" water I loathe. I even have a bromine-laden, thyroid-disrupting hot tub I frequent. So simply do the best you can with your circumstances. You need to be a realist. You cannot live in a bubble or freak out. You can, however, be proactive and minimize as best you can, where you can. It is a matter of choice.

Again, just drink water.

Perhaps you really enjoy Vitamin Water or Splenda infused flavored water. I'll never touch that stuff. Why should I or you?

It doesn't matter to me that my favorite athlete drinks a particular manufactured, water-based, highly marketed beverage. On television, it really seems that he/she enjoys it, so I don't drink it so that the company can send them another case.

For some time, I have been recommending tea and herbal teas. Unless you live in a box, you already know that tea is good for you. The standard for a long time has been green tea. The reason that it is touted is because of the antioxidant polyphenols. The major polyphenols in tea are flavonoids, and the most common in tea being catechins and epigallocatechin gallate (EGCG). I say this understanding that while we may think we understand tea and its constituents fully, I laugh to think that we feel we know it all. I am of the resolve that tea is *still* a mystery to us. The beauty of it is that we do not need to understand tea we simply need to drink it!

The benefits of tea(s) herbal or otherwise are numerous: fights bacteria, fights fungus, fights virus, assists in blood sugar maintenance.

But forget all that. Remember simply that tea is good for you. Plain and simple. In the Normal Diet, you should drink tea. Obviously, you make tea with water. So two birds with one stone. Water and life-enhancing green tea is a staple for me.

Well, what about black tea? And hasn't white tea been shown to be even better than both of them? Well, yes, arguably, you would be correct. I have heard it said that decaf tea is worse than regular tea as chemicals are used to strip the caffeine off. So what should you do?

I myself drink tea, whether hot, cold, regular, or decaf virtually every day. A better statement is that I continue to consume tea consistently over the past many decades. Green tea is my basic go-to, yet I also include various herbal teas as well. Ashwagandha, lemon balm, raspberry, dandelion, licorice, nettle leaf, chamomile, echinacea, etc. I prefer all my teas to be organic, which is simple enough to obtain. At this very moment, I am having a turmeric blend.

Don't add or adulterate your tea. Save it for another area that is worthy of going nuts with, like ice cream. Go plain. You'll get used to and love it. If you want to use other teas, then do it. I really enjoy Earl Grey tea as well.

When I was young, my grandmother instilled in me a love and respect for tea. When I think of her, I generally picture her with a cup of tea nearby and usually some toast. I also remember how she used to add milk and sugar to her tea, so I did also. I did this for many years. I didn't know any better. Now I do.

My grandmother would also place a lukewarm tea bag on our eyes if we had an infection or styes. This has worked well over the years for me, my family, and my patients. It is what her mother did and her mother before that.

Tea is natures medicine. Powerful at that. Once you add other things to it, I feel you begin to degrade the healing abilities that reside within. Sugar is a huge no-no. Don't do it.

For some, they say they cannot do without sugar or honey for that matter. It is in your best interest to avoid sugar in general and especially in your tea.

Children benefit the same way as adults from consuming tea on a regular basis. I started having my daughters boil water and make tea for me when they were old enough to do so. I would invite them to take sips of it from time to time.

Gradually, they began to like it. During the colder months, I would bring a large cup of tea to the bus stop. We would all huddle around the only form of heat and play "touch the tea." We would each take turns holding and then sipping the hot tea for warmth.

Little did they know, I was indoctrinating them. My son, on the other hand, wasn't so receptive. However, with gentle encouraging and seeing everyone else in the family drinking tea regularly, he began to take sips. Now he drinks tea. I pray they all will consume plain teas their whole life.

Yes, we may have coffee or less-than-desirable beverages, but through it all, we drink tea. That's what we do, and that is what you may want to consider doing as well.

Now matcha green tea is purported to be one of the strongest teas. Earlier, I had mentioned that tea is beneficial due to the polyphenols. Matcha green tea is said to have more EGCGs than other green teas.

All this said, just drink tea; that is the overall point. Clean, self-brewed, no sugar. Keep it simple. Remember, we are slowly introducing those items into your lifestyle that enhance and eliminating those that hinder your health. Adding tea is easy.

Back to basic water consumption. If you feel you are having trouble simply drinking plain water, may I encourage you to add fresh slice(s) of lemon or limes. These are healing in their own right in many ways. Sometimes I have both. So refreshing.

During the summer months, I have been known to add freshly squeezed lemons and splash of apple cider vinegar to water. Again, refreshing, clean, and healing.

Allow me to conclude this *whole water thing* by expressing that being intentional and consistent with water intake is the springboard to greater overall health. We spend so much time, money, and effort seeking out the Holy Grail of it all when the answer in large part lies freely before us.

Simply drink more water.

All of our body systems upregulate with proper hydration. Think about it. When you drink clean water, your health improves beginning that very moment. If you take away nothing else from this material, please consider maintaining a daily intake of water. You will be glad you did!

5

AM Basic Training

Where in the world do we start the nuts-and-bolts discussion of the Normal Diet? Truth is, I believe we already did… and then some as mindset about our health needs to precede what we put in our mouths. The real issue is that most want some sort of scheduled plan to follow, and while that may assist in the application of the Normal Diet, what we want is more of a *sense* to what you should be doing and just let it flow already. Does that seem rationale to you? I hope it does. By now, you should know that the Normal Diet consists of maximizing real food and minimizing fake food.

While seemingly obvious, this is simply the most important statement I will make as it pertains to your health. As such, it bears repeating often, and so I shall. When you consume *real* food, your health improves. When you ingest *fake* food, your health declines.

Such a statement used to be rudimentary whereas these days, it's borderline revolutionary. Unless you decide here and now to become intentional about what you put into your body, you will find that most that go in your tank will be fabricated by science, a pseudo-food.

We will cover this more as we work through it all. For now, let's pull into focus actionable steps to get our health moving in the right direction. So what is the very first step?

That's what you truly want to know. I know this because that's what each of us desire-to know "my" next step. Right?

Is the first step the same step for everyone? This is where we could potentially fall into a trap. Is the Normal Diet just another book that is here today gone tomorrow? If so, then we easily put something together that resembles the same hierarchical flow chart created by all the others who have come before us. This isn't that type of program.

To be clear, the Normal Diet is more of an *understanding of principles* that you come to see as a truth that anchors inside your heart *before* it manifests in your physical actionable world. Does that sound too new age and transcendental? It shouldn't but it kinda does—so let's simply agree that what we are looking for first and foremost is an *inner shift* wherein you shake off the old *you* and have this guttural yearning to simply do better, feel better, be better, and generally mature in understanding your nutritional needs as the years move along.

Through it all, the basics will always be the basics. These essentials will be a safe harbor for you. The basics will not let you down; in fact, these simple truths will guide you back to the path you really want to be on.

Perhaps the simplest place to start is with fluid intake. That is why we covered water before jumping in here. No matter how lousy you feel—whether its achy joint pain, autoimmune flair, brain fog, constipation, infection, rash, headaches, fatigue, anger, and everything else that afflicts us, basic training always, and I mean always includes water. Start here and we can go anywhere else. Skip this step at your own peril.

If, when, once you understand, agree to and implement "the whole water thing," then what comes next exactly? Simply put, what comes next is already being answered in your head even before I say it. You are now turning your own attention to two items. Those two areas are (1) what you know you need to *stop*, stop doing—

stop eating, stop drinking. And (2) what you already know you need to *begin*, begin doing—begin eating and/or begin drinking. If you think this is double talk, then you haven't been following along really. This is where the rubber hits the road. You *innately* know what you need to stop and what you need to start. I am not saying you are yet willing to follow through and actually start. I am simply being frank by maturely revealing the undeniable truth that you already have a clear understanding of what you need to face. Can we agree to that at least?

So that said, the next step in the Normal Diet "plan" is simply not to go freak out. After fluid uptake and before anything else, you need to develop a clear understanding that henceforth, we will *gently* and *sequentially* achieve forward momentum by addressing the issue(s) that are the easiest for you to handle…not the hardest. Address the "low-hanging fruit"—yes, pun intended again.

Sequential implementation of the changes you need to make thereby leading to upregulation of your overall health may be a new approach yet understand it for what it is—a gentle path forward that is sustainable for each and every one of us no matter where this material finds you.

For many, if not most, a good place to give initial attention to begins with the nurturing of yourself during the morning routines you have. Yes, what you do in the morning might drastically need to change yet set that aside for now and for the next couple days just take stock of what you actually do currently, whether right or wrong.

Feel free to take a week and write down what is a typical morning for you, what you do, what you eat, drink, etc. Simply gather data. Then analyze this information. You might surprise yourself if you look at it all as an active observer. Just watch yourself and see what you're actually doing versus what you think you are doing. Do not judge. This is a natural starting point; understand where you want to go yet know what we are beginning with.

Once we kinda know our own personal patterns, then we begin to gently modify...something. Perhaps your morning assessment reveals you actually are drinking a pot of coffee and tablespoons of sugar. Do we get rid of the coffee altogether, or do we begin by drinking a half glass of water while the coffee is brewing? That's rational and easy enough, isn't it? Yes, it is and this is our mindset all along the journey with our own normal diets. Even if you just don't feel like doing it, simply do so on the smallest level that is acceptable for you; start with a sip of water, and before you know it, you won't be able to do without it.

Now as far as breakfast, I get it that we typically have a small window to consume something. So let's not make breakfast so complicated. However, you should make it nutritious. From my perspective on the matter, while we are led to believe that breakfast is the most important meal of the day, it shouldn't be the biggest, fattiest meal of the day. I perceive the AM hours should offer up easily assimilated nutritional rich items that do not overload your system right out of the gate. If you wake up and have sausage, doughnuts, and bagels, you can best be sure that if you're over forty, you'll be suffering with those decisions almost immediately...and for a couple days thereafter. While I enjoy avocado toast, the fat/bread overload combination isn't an everyday-type thing.

No matter where you turn, you could and do find opposing views to all things dietary-related. I am simply asking you to consider that the AM time frame sets the tone for the rest of the day and days ahead. Let's gently approach this with nutrients that easily provide for the body without an all-out assault, stress, and endocrine shock.

For now, but perhaps not forever, may I recommend a blended smoothie of sorts to feed you—to wake up the furnace inside. These concoctions do not need to impress anyone. They really do not even need to taste good, but that's a bonus. My smoothies are much different now then what they used to be.

When I first transitioned to an AM smoothie routine, I most certainly had the base liquid as milk or, for that matter, light cream. I would add fruit that was going rotten in the corner of the kitchen that my then very young children would not eat. So that's really how I started…as the "clean-up man." I was the last hope of certain food items to be eaten; otherwise, they were being thrown out. That's true, and it makes me laugh to think about it. Whichever fruit was bruised and battered ended up in my morning smoothies—hysterical.

Nowadays, my base liquid is typically water. That may not sound thrilling, but that's the truth of it. I do use almond milk or coconut water on occasion, however, and yes, I've been still known to put in some light or heavy cream. I don't feel dairy is actually that fantastic of a decision, yet I am simply telling you what normal people do on a normal diet.

Increasingly, my morning shakes have had more of what I would consider a detoxification application. What does that mean exactly? Well, it means that I have kinda set taste aside in hopes of blending together whatever it takes to clean out some garbage I myself created within me.

In a base of water with protein plant powder scoops I typically add frozen blueberries, which are usually wild grown. These are readily available in virtually all stores so don't think it is difficult. I also have been adding in a pinch of curcumin/turmeric powder, small half teaspoon of fiber, Hawaiian spirulina powder, barley grass or barley grass *juice* powder, wheatgrass. I do still look for the bruised fruit as my now adult children still abhor the slightest imperfection. Maybe one day, it's half a banana. Another day, sliced mango, apple, pear, etc.

I blend this together and drink slowly over about twenty minutes or so. I have and do use cilantro. I have put in ginger in my smoothies as well as about anything else you could imagine. Tomatoes, carrots, celery are fair game also. I only use little bits of different things as not to overwhelm.

People ask me about chia. I do use chia. I do put protein oats, flax, and everything and anything I feel that I (a) want or (b) my body needs. Not all together—simply at different intervals. Maybe

I go through "a round" of more veggie smoothies for a couple weeks and then a detox-type concoction for many weeks and then onto a more fruit-filled smoothie. If we don't change it all up, we would be missing the point of getting a wide variety of healthy nutrients into our bodies.

If you want to add in some orange slices, go ahead. The point to AM basic training is to keep it simple while getting good nutrients into the tank out of the gate. I will be candid in that sometimes, such a simple breakfast leaves me hungry not long after. I have been known to either add more plant protein powders, a scoop of coconut oil, olive oil, or even avocado.

Earlier stating that you should avoid heavy oils and fats and then tell you that I have been known to do just that seems almost hypocritical here. I am simply telling you that keeping breakfast clean for a while, you will eventually come to understand how your body feels, reacts, responds to your choices. You can retool from there. When I now know that the next time I will be able to grab something to eat is extended, I will add something additional to sustain and get me through.

By and large, I recommend Standard Process Complete as my product of choice for a couple scoops of plant-based powder, which I add to my smoothies. SP complete is whole food not fake food. It contains a base of whey, flax, rice proteins, brussels sprouts, buckwheat, alfalfa, lecithin, inositol, grapeseed extract, and carrot. There is more but you get the point. It is food. Not imitation.

Some would say whey is no good. Others might ask if gluten is in the powder. It's mostly organic but maybe not all organic is that a problem? Look, I love Standard Process products. I don't think you can find better and touting that takes a lot for me to say. I was introduced to Standard Process when I was ten years old, and I have been consistently relying on them since.

Could something in their whole food or herbal line not meet up to your scrutiny in some fashion? Probably but that's not the issue. The real issue is that what your doing is not really working that well, so let's drop the shoulders, lower your defenses, and let's simply acquire *real food*—whether powder form or otherwise—and start ingesting.

Sometimes I simply take plant-based food powder and keep it dry in a shaker cup and drink it in between regular meals as I feel needed. As I get older, I simply do not want to starve, yet I do not want to feel bloated and regretful of what I ate or even overate. Simply something to satisfy. It's basic, yet sometimes this is just what you may require.

I have heard it said that in order to live longer and healthier, you may want to consider eating less food and consuming more happiness. Much truth here.

This highlights the fact that not every meal needs to be a major endeavor. In fact, for some, the initial smoothie idea may be what you feel you need to do for three "meals" per day for a week or maybe two. Almost like a "quick start." I use my smoothies to reset myself after a weekend where my intake did not live up to my own standards. I am so happy to get that Monday morning shake in me, and should I need, I'll have another for lunch. Again, not every single time just when I know I need a break and a restart.

But after water and nutrient-dense smoothie, where do we go? Should basic training jump right to protein? Yes and no. We can get to that in a little bit. Before we go further, we need to acknowledge that while we may have *added* something, I believe we need to address the *removal* of something. That *thing* is sugar.

The Normal Diet hinges on reducing the body's burden generally. Water and various smoothies help to cleanse, heal, remove, unburden glands, organs, and tissues but why do that if you're simply slamming it with garbage and sugar right thereafter. You are creating your own vicious cycle and fostering "dis-ease" down the road.

If we just discussed what we could simply and sequentially add maybe—just maybe—we look to sequentially remove sugar. This doesn't have to be complete cessation at this point; let's just consider where you can do less.

Do you really need sugar-laden tea or coffee as soon as your feet hit the ground? Maybe now you do, but if you keep doing this decade after decade, you won't have feet to hit the ground with one day. Ouch—that's harsh, and it's reality for thousands of people.

I just read recently that some one hundred thousand people died from diabetes in the past year. That number pretty much applied to the year before as well. How many more hundreds of thousands didn't pass away yet are on the verge of having tissue amputated? Geez, I don't even want to discuss this, yet it could be a reality for any one of us if we do not reign in self and follow a better path. The Normal Diet is that better path.

Basic training afternoon and PM basic training will be discussed, yet you need to understand what we covered here thus far. Keep it simple. Let's get results; let's not get confused. It's not all as difficult as we want to pretend it is.

From time to time, I will be asked if the sugar that naturally occurs in fruit, is also a type of sugar to avoid. The short answer would appear to be yes from a sugar standpoint and its effect on blood sugar levels shortly after consumption.

Look, I love fruit and you love fruit. God made fruit. Fruit fits the premise of "if God made it, eat it" viewpoint. Are their exceptions? I bet there is, but why worry about that—let's simply agree that fresh fruit is healthy and leads to better satisfaction overall.

I would ask that we perhaps reduce or limit fruits in the context that in the beginning I am guessing that whether appropriately or inappropriately that by and large you are having way too much sugars in all its many forms.

So while it would to be better to skip all the garbage sugars and stick with fresh fruits, if we need to cut back just a little in all departments temporarily to have forward momentum, then I am not against it.

One way to scientifically evaluate the amount of sugars coursing through your veins is to simply purchase a basic glucometer from the local store. This is common for someone who has diabetes to consider, yet even if you don't, or don't want to end up with an elevated sugar problem, why not see what your blood sugars are from time to time.

From my own experience, it is truly eye opening to take your blood levels first thing in the morning and already be elevated. Then consume an all-out fruit smoothie and have those blood sugars shoot even higher wondering the whole time if something is really wrong. It makes you change your ways and change them fast!

Candidly as I have grown older, I can see just how sensitive my body has become to various food groups generally yet sugar specifically. This is a common occurrence for most if not all. Recognizing this truth that it is goes a long way in maintaining health through our later years.

I do *not* want to burn my body out. Neither do you.

If you think sugar doesn't have an immediate impact on your physiological function, you are grossly mistaken.

Go ahead and check your radial pulse. That's what you feel at the level of your wrist. Take the next sixty seconds and see how many beats you feel. Write that number down. At rest, my hope it's about sixty to seventy beats per minute or thereabouts.

Now go ahead and take some sugar in your mouth. Maybe a piece of candy like a yummy Jolly Rancher would do. After a minute or so of enjoying this sugary delight of your choice, go back and once again feel the pulse and see how many beats the next sixty seconds brings.

I can virtually guarantee that your pulse rate elevates at least five or more. Maybe much more depending on your level of health.

Many years ago, when I did this, I was quite surprised at the elevated pulse that occurred.

Now as far as protein goes, we have made it way too complicated, and I aim to correct that now. Eating protein is as *essential* as is clearly appropriate fats and carbohydrates.

You need protein. It is this simple.

The individual who needs to check all the boxes might press me and inquire as to how much protein they need or *should* consume in a day. Once that's answered, you can bet the discussion turns to how much at one sitting, what types, what forms as in solids, liquids.

Some may ask at what time(s) should they eat protein. Is more protein in the morning better than at night? Should you take liquid protein within thirty minutes post-workout or maybe set an alarm to wake you up during the night for a couple scoops of nut butters.

My answer to all these questions and more usually is, "How should I know"?

I do feel that at a minimum 0.5 gram to 1 gram per pound of body weight *desired* should at the very least be considered taken in through the course of a day if you want to make some changes in bodily tone.

For example, if someone who weighs 240 lb. desires to lean out to around 200 lb., then try and target protein in a range from 100 to 200 grams per day. Feel it out. Experiment within this range. Your body will tell you in some way. This is not weird; it's just the way it is.

Do not overthink this. Just eat protein in some fashion. It is not difficult, but it will take intention. A smoothie can be 30 grams to 50 grams of protein simply by switching in and out ingredients.

If you boil some eggs and add that into the mix along with legumes, nuts, and the standby poultry, fish and beef you will hit your mark and really enjoy yourself. If you stick to liverwurst and pork roll, I think that's a mistake as it's a wide range of nutrients that we need to ingest to have various building blocks leading to health and vitality.

I laugh to think how many times I am pushed back on when discussing a patients need to increase protein intake or at the very least balance their consumption proportionately to their current fats or carbohydrate levels.

People generally think if they take in too much protein, they will burn out their kidneys. I really hear that, and while a rare condition, I suppose that can and perhaps has happened. What's more common is burning out kidneys and every other gland, organ, and tissue from sugar.

So let's not pretend here, shall we?

The deal with asking you to consider an AM smoothie is predicated on that so many reading this have bodies that simply need a break from the abuse and burden placed on it. To also unburden stress on the body, you may want to consider the concept of reducing food intake or *fasting* at certain times. The topic of fasting itself has been the focus of volumes of books and material itself. I perceive intermittent fasting has significant benefit when applied correctly and appropriately on a case-by-case basis.

Recently, a fifty-four-year-old, heavy-set, nonathletic, borderline diabetic male told me he was scared that he had to fast for his blood work.

Guess what happened?

He stated that he "surprisingly felt great" not eating past 7:00 PM. Because of his schedule, he couldn't get to the blood draw lab until after 11:00 AM the following day, then he had an earlier lunch. That's some fifteen hours of "time-out" right there. He didn't crash, faint, or otherwise.

This person then said, "I am beginning to think that what I eat is having an effect on the way I feel." I would have laughed out loud if this person wasn't so deadpan serious.

He was correct in that he doesn't feel that good because what he eats isn't that good. The body doesn't forget! The decades of poor nutritional intake has led to his current state on declining health albeit a slower descent than many.

The light went on. I saw the flicker of understanding that he wants to, needs to change.

This person then asked if (1) can he fast like that again, and if so when, how long, how often, etc., and (2) he asked if he could replace his morning cereal, bagels, yogurts with scrambled eggs for the next week or so.

The answer to the first was, let's go slow here. The answer to the second is absolutely, stay on just eggs for a month if you like, and let's see what happens.

I can hear the egg haters now. One group laments the high cholesterols contained within…that's a joke, and the other group protests as eggs could be a more source of food allergy. Maybe much truth on the second one there, but can we agree for now that maybe, just maybe, organic eggs could potentially be better than, let's say, the dozen doughnuts being consumed each week?

Eat protein. Enough said.

Now as we pull to the close of the Normal Diet AM basic training discussion, know that it may take a little while to change those poor, long-standing morning habits. If you find yourself with chocolate all over your face from the icing atop a Boston cream donut you slammed down, do not despair! All you need to do is get back to what you know you should be doing.

What is that exactly?

Well, my dear reader, for now, allow the launch to be in the form of a highly nutritious and extremely tasty smoothie concoction. Have fun with this. I know you will!

6

Food Fabrication

In case you haven't heard by now, much of what is consumed is not really food at all. Much of the *food* is better described as *food like stuff*. We eat more scientifically engineered consumable product than we do actual God-made food.

The fact is that you cannot escape fake food unless you live on an island, and even there, McDonald's is petitioning the zoning hearing board to allow a variance for its first ever sail through line! Industrialized food has made its way to the farthest reaches of the globe. This is hailed as perhaps one of the greatest achievements of modernism. It is far from it. Why you ask? Let's get to that.

Nowadays the vast majority of producers in the plant kingdom are turning to genetically modified organisms, aka GMOs. The GMOs are scientifically altered organisms; for the sake of this conversation, let's call it seeds that have their genes modified, made to withstand and be resistant against diseases, insects, and herbicides, hopefully leading to greater crop yields.

Some say this allows for less chemicals to be sprayed on fields as well as less tilling on the land, saving the farmers time and money. Perhaps the optimistic aspect of greater yields per acre could mean less food prices as more food is produced, yet I cannot say anyone has seen food prices drop at all.

Some also say that as a result of reduced spraying, less is running off into streams and other water sources. If I was a farmer, I would want something that would allow for better outcomes and be less work for me. That's normal. Who wouldn't like to make more money and work less these days?

I spoke with a fourth-generation corn and bean farmer on this topic. It went something like this: "Hey, Dan, do you guys use those GMO seeds?"

Dan responded, "You mean roundup ready seeds? Yeah, I use them, they are great. I don't have to go back and spray the fields as often. So I can try and catch up on everything else I have been falling behind on, one of them is sleep!"

So I cannot blame our farmers one bit. These guys are giving their lives day in and day out to deliver the goods. I could probably have told him the reasons he needed to stop using these *frankenseeds*, yet I believe it would have fallen on gentle yet deaf ears. Again, I do not fault him.

I could have discussed with him, or anyone for that matter, that while GMO crops promised greater yields, it has delivered at best negligible gains. In addition, the use of herbicides have not diminished! Glyphosate, the active ingredient in most popular herbicides, is arguably slowly killing humans and other life forms. That is not solely my belief. Dr. Stephanie Seneff who is an MIT researcher has studied glyphosate for about ten years. I can only imagine the push back and the suppression of her assertion that glyphosate is behind increased autism, diabetes, cancers, allergies, and other disease. *Ugh* is all I can say.

As far as corporate producers go, I could have given Dan an impassioned "save the plant from evil conglomerate control of the world's food supply" pleading, which I also believe is happening before our eyes, yet again, our local independent farmers are not public enemy number 1. No, sir, they are our friends, our neighbors, who are trying to do their jobs and callings as best they know how. Imagine someone telling you that your occupation is leading to all diseases on a grand scale.

I could have directed Dan to watch the movie, *Food, Inc.* or have given him a copy of *Omnivore's Dilemma* both by Michael Pollan, which is simply a must-watch and a must-read from my perspective.

I could have gone on and on yet for the moment, for Dan, he just wants to take a break and make more money *for* and spend time *with* his family. One or two less passes across hundreds of acres each growing season is huge. Maybe he would only have to work a half day on Sundays. Get my point? I can't fault him. He's kind. He works hard as his father and his father's father before him did. It doesn't make these GMO's any better for him you or me. It's just the way he sees it from his perspective. I get it.

With the advent of a company's ability to now manufacture genetically modified strains of seed as in soy or corn comes patents and guaranteed-protection status. When the farmers purchase the seeds from, let's say, Cargill or Monsanto, they are not just buying corn seed; they are buying *their* corn seed, which comes with a catch or two. The seeds are only good for one growing season, after which, you keep going back each year to buy them. Also, at any time, these companies can come in and test your corn to see if you are wrongly using their genetically manufactured product. If so, you're screwed. Problem is that cross pollination among fields is affecting the natural crops. It is messy and getting worse. Will we even have natural heirloom produce left in the next decade? Nobody can, or should I say want to, address this question.

If you are a person of faith, you cannot help but feel that prophecy is coming to fruition as it appears at some point in the future, there will be a controller of the worlds food supply as written in Revelation. Topic of another book, I suppose.

If you go on the computer and search for "Millions against Monsanto," you will quickly understand just how dire the situation has become. As a side note, the relationship between agribusiness and pharmaceutical industry is now complete since the Bayer Monsanto merger. I want to be optimistic, I really do, yet I just do not see how this and other unholy alliances are working toward the betterment of the human race.

Producers of genetically modified organism (GMO) products are clearly out to make as much profit as they can make. We need to remember that. I perceive that we are desiring to believe, no, maybe it is more like being sold the notion that Monsanto has a more altruistic reason—that being hunger.

In 2010, Monsanto was chosen as company of the year by Forbes magazine. Such a title given to this company seems bizarre. Even more strange is that, generally, Americans know very little about GMOs and the impact it most certainly will have. I am rather optimistic person, yet I am not so sure this GMO freight train will be stopped.

Many issues surround the GMO effect from economic to physiologic. Perhaps a topic I am not well equipped to fully argue, yet I do know that once again utilizing the lost art of common sense this does not end well. The GMO seeds are designed with a self-limiting component inherent to it. This only allows for one season of germination. This requires the farmer to keep coming back to the company and purchasing their products year after year.

Let me be clear: I am not against corporate profits, and neither should you. It is not a "bad company" in the profit-making sense; it is a view that such practices of genetically modifying seeds are fundamentally an abomination of nature with significant consequences looming on the horizon. As if there wasn't enough to deal with already, it may be the case that genetically modified and created food will result in more devastation than it pretends to do otherwise. To keep an open mind to the benefits of GMOs, I have done my best to find in favor for it. I haven't. In fact, I believe the evidence is insurmountable against it.

Farmers who have elected to not use GMO seeds are finding their crops cross-contaminated by farmers that do. The end result is them being sued for using a GMO product without paying for it. Absurd. They should be suing Monsanto for contamination.

Clearly, I am sharing the truth of the matter combined with a personal aggravated opine here, yet it is my name on the cover, so occasionally, I feel I am able to take literary license. I am not an attorney. I am simply an observer of what looks to be an ever-increasing stranglehold on what is our God-given right—that being to eat what the Earth provides to sustain us. Not what we are judicially subject to from corporations or courts. Absurd. These are the days in which we find ourselves.

The South African advertising standards authority found Monsanto guilty of falsely claiming that no negative reactions have been associated with genetically modified food. This was back in 2007. How much more issues have been swept under the rug in the years since? One can only ponder.

I suspect we will be hearing more about negative effects from these scientifically created foods. It may be sudden reactions; however, my feeling is that it will be a generational type of effect. Again, the understandable cross-contamination that was mentioned and the resultant hybrids may be leading to potentially genetically harmful DNA-changing mishap of the next generation(s).

Yes, I am saying that there exists the very real possibility that consumption of GMOs could, or more to the point *will* lead to a whole generation of affected individuals. Our children and grandchildren.

What about solving hunger? Doesn't genetically altered food have more to offer? Won't we be living in a land of plenty from now on with enough to go around? Not quite. Turns out that genetically modified soy has 20 percent less yield than traditional soy and up to 100 percent failure of cotton crops in India. I should say that was some time ago. So it is not a given that GMOs will deliver on their promise in this regard.

I suppose we could address the downsides apart from future health crisis GMOs may cause. A USDA and University of Georgia study found that using GMO cotton in the US can result in a drop in income of up to 40 percent. How can this be? It is. We just haven't heard about it like we should have.

The discussion I had with a local farmer that I mentioned earlier was perhaps the single bright spot in this whole confusing mess. The farmer could have a little bit easier of a time. Or so it seems. With fewer crops and less income, who wins?

The notion of less pesticide use is also smoke and mirrors. Turns out that USDA data demonstrates a rise in pesticide usage by some 50 million pounds from 1996 to 2003. Also, the use of glyphosate doesn't make anyone feel safe. As stated earlier, this is a known carcinogen and physiological disrupter. Not surprisingly, use of this toxin has increased by fifteen times more during 1994 to 2005 to address the rise of superweeds, which have become resistant to this and other herbicides. Takes more to kill them. Sound familiar? Antibiotics come to mind.

So after all this discussion, what should we conclude? I surmise that we do our best to avoid any and all GMO foods. This begs the question of, "How do you know if it is or isn't?" Truth is, this just isn't clear anymore. Seeking out non-GMO sources and organic foods should give us a leg up in the short run. However, with inflation skyrocketing in all areas this is not economically, aka family, budget friendly in the least.

That said, the true cost could potentially be our health decades down the road if we simply follow the herd. Time will tell.

I'll admit that fake food can taste really good at times, especially when you are "starving." The short-term pleasure is much different from the joy and fortitude your body would derive from God-made food items that actually nourish our bodies.

Who doesn't like Jolly Ranchers? As a kid, I couldn't ever turn one away if it was offered. That sweet taste was incredible, especially the watermelon ones. Could we exist or thrive solely on Jolly Ranchers? Of course not, that's ludicrous.

In this awkward analogy, it is as if we, ourselves, are living on Jolly Rancher–type food products that for all intents and purpose appear pleasing to the eye, delightful to the palate, but little if nothing more. The mind/body connection recognizes these edible products and in it goes. The body is then challenged to rummage through and make use of what little it has been given to thrive. Repeated behavior of withholding body-building nutrients from the body can only lead to one thing, poor health, sickness, suffering, and premature death.

The food fabricators may be enriching their products to comply with the generally accepted recommended daily allowance (RDA) criteria that exists today, but I am not so sure that we benefit as consumers. In fact, I am being polite. I believe we have no benefit whatsoever by regularly consuming "enriched" vitamin or mineral sprinkled fake food sources that lack all the naturally occurring enzymes and cofactors that exist in the natural state. Enhanced, enriched, or even pressed into a supplement, fabricated anything is just not the best choice for the body whether human, dog, fish, or bird.

Yes, clearly, the products we are offered are edible. Less apparent is the nutritional benefit obtained for long-term growth, maintenance, and vitality. Is it a stretch to say our food is making us sick? It is pretty clear the food you are eating can either make you healthier or make you sicker, bite by bite and sip by sip.

I can think of many specific fake food products and their manufactures, but let's keep our discussion more general as to not offend even though the way we have been duped is itself utterly offensive. Our disease-ravaged society should be offended to the point of revolting against such flagrant disregard for human health and longevity. We are not yet to that point on a mass scale. When we are, I envision companies that are "too big to fail" failing or completely changing altogether.

In the general sense, our snacks are one of the greatest offenders to proper nutrition. What exactly is pork rinds anyway? What about cheese puffs?

When people generally shop, they tend to look at the front of the packaging. On the front, you see happy, smiling, satisfied faces. On the back label, you see the nutritional ingredients or, in our discussion, lack thereof.

The label themselves may tell you *what's* in the item, yet please understand it doesn't tell you how it was prepared, or should I say *fabricated*. This is worth really thinking about for a minute. Give thought to just how the item you hold in your hand was made. Set aside the genetically altered process for the moment and let's just say an apple is an apple, but how many different ways can one make applesauce? I would think the simplest version is crushing one or more apples together until reaching the desired consistency. I say this in jest but, on the other end of the spectrum, is a possible version of applesauce that has gone through such cooking/processing and added ingredients and preservatives that make it more like an *idea* of what applesauce is rather than a tried-and-true *apple, which is sauced.* The better the applesauce taste, you can be pretty sure it went through a lot of processing.

On the front, you see bold lettering indicating the special fortification, the health endorsements, and such. On the back, you generally have a challenging time pronouncing the ingredients, all twenty-five of them.

Remember when our biggest concern was salt intake? Oh, the glory days of yore. To only be worried about sodium again would be a blessing.

If I were to summarize what we discussed here this chapter, it would be along the lines of "If God made it, then eat it. If mankind made it, try not to eat it, and if your spouse made it, then you had better eat it…"

7

The Pig-Out

I have done it. You have done it. My bet is that it will happen again when you least expect it. At any given time on any given day, and despite your best-laid plans. Despite all your mental stamina. Despite all hypnotic safeguards or subliminal messages, you will inevitably have a moment (or two) of weakness where you find your-self, well, just plain *pigging out*.

Kevin is a forty-two-year-old father of two. Avid cyclist. He first came to my clinic for true wellness care. Kevin is an otherwise healthy individual wanting to maintain and further his wellbeing. We retooled his dietary intake to better reflect his specific needs. We added specific foods at specific times based on his work, family, and exercise routines. Timing his intake of food was what made a big difference for him.

One afternoon, I got a phone call from him saying it was important to speak to me. He was calm but direct when he told me that for several weeks, he was having incredible cravings for sweets like he has never had before. He couldn't get enough. Before he fully blew his program and improvements to date, he wanted to see what we could do to get him back on the right path.

Now pigging out for each of us is a bit different. For Kevin, it was a sudden and overwhelming sweet-tooth type of thing. For some, it could be a bag of trail mix. For others, maybe yams, corn on the cob, or pickled beets. You just can't always predict what it will be. While some cravings are highly specific, the pig-out is more generalized.

I have seen it endless times where my patients would say something like "I just couldn't stop." When discussed further, you hear that they started with a carrot, proceeded to spoonsful of yogurt, then the leftover chicken dipped into mayo, and then finished up with a peanut butter and jelly on crackers, all while drinking milk from the bottle never shutting the Frigidaire door the entire time.

The point being that the pig-out is not as specific as a craving. Let me retract that slightly and state that the person is craving something that *perhaps* their conscious mind just doesn't seem to know what it is.

In the pig-out, you generally keep consuming until the point of being somewhat sick, disgusted, and feeling more than a bit guilty. The problem is that the pig-out is usually over before you know it.

The pig-out does more than just blindside all our best intentions and efforts it demoralizes us. And that, my dear friends, is the crux of it all—how we *feel* as we stand in the destructive aftermath of our actions either fosters new resolve or, like many, if not most, jumping ship altogether and pretending the "diet" didn't work. Many occasions, the patients I treat come in with their heads hung low, declaring that they failed or begging for forgiveness, something along those lines.

I am not the one to be absolving people in the least. I will listen and assist in guiding them back to where we both know they want to go. But the pig-out needs to be addressed or at least better understood so that it doesn't completely stop the progress being made. Momentum is everything.

Yes, the pig-out *feels good* while it is occurring, albeit very brief, but the mental anguish and self-deprecation is never worth it in hindsight.

The more individuals I see that are involved with an exclusionary diet program, the higher the odds of them succumbing to the pig-out. Yes, even those die-hard Atkins fans fall prey to the pig-out. For the extreme Atkins eater, the initial onslaught of all the bacon, blue cheese, buffalo wings you can handle sounds fabulous, at least for a season. In these cases, the pig-out is pasta, breads, bagels, and doughnuts!

As an aside, I perceive Dr. Atkins as a genius of an individual. He bucked the norm and really stuck his neck out to get the lower-carbohydrate lifestyle heading in the right direction. Is it in line with the Normal Diet? Not necessarily, but neither is a no-fat diet. Neither is a vegetarian diet. Neither is any diet that specifically excludes a macro or micronutrient.

Now getting back to the pig-out. It is going to happen, so why not accept as much and lean into it rather than being shocked that it could and will occur. Perhaps then we can better handle what happens next. So *plan* for the pig-out—in fact, I support as much from time to time! For me, personally, it happens usually around holidays and birthdays. Guess what, I am going to pass away one day anyway. A few well-placed pig-outs won't make that much of a difference.

A word of caution as if you make every day a pig-out day, then we have a problem. In America, every day tends to be a pig-out day and that's what has us in the health crisis we find ourselves in! The planned pig-outs are one thing while the sustained pig-outs are quite another.

Well, how often can you have a pig-out day and still be staying on task? Good question with no easy answer. The hard-line answer is that we shouldn't have a pig-out event at all. The realistic way to answer is to simply acknowledge that the nature of humankind is such that as sure as we breath these events will occur.

To some, this may seem like a cop-out. Maybe this is a hypocritical way to rationalize our shortcomings, our blunders, and perhaps our lack of character. Really? Is that true? Maybe the critical person who takes this view is the knuckle head themselves. If you recall "To err is human."

Let's get one thing straight: No one, not one person, young or old, male, or female, wants to fail. This doesn't just pertain to our health and nutritional intake. We are talking about life, our visions, our dreams, and goals.

So when we talk specifically about the nutrition for our bodies, it must understand that each one of us started with certain desires and aspirations that we perceive as worthy.

Using the logical mind, we didn't even need to consider the pig-out type event at the start. And that by and large is the fundamental mistake virtually everyone makes.

The feeding frenzy has little to do with logic at all. It must do more so with feelings, emotions, and hormones.

Now it isn't just the negative emotions that can spawn an unstoppable eating tsunami; it is also the positive emotions. Sure, getting dumped in a relationship would be a classic example. "Drowning your sorrows" in food or beverages for that matter, is not a new concept. It sure is a good excuse, though, isn't it? It certainly derails a good, clean start. If not reeled in, it leads to just another failed attempt that does little to further our health or self-esteem.

However, a sudden rush of a good and beneficial emotional state of being can get you off the path as well except your having such a good time that you don't recognize it until you find yourself two steps back…again.

Case in point, you have been exercising, getting proper rest, maybe lost a few pounds of water weight, got a nice compliment or two. You are feeling good.

Maybe you just completed your first 5K run for fun. Maybe you're just feeling more energy and more relaxed.

It is at a heightened sense of "I am doing so good" that many expose their Achilles's heel. Believe me, we all have them.

Suddenly, the defenses are pierced with the "I have been doing great, I deserve this" thought pattern. Dangerous thinking. Typically ends with an antacid and a day or more of feeling off both mentally and physically.

Now the hormone discussion is nothing to slight. However, it does go beyond the scope of what we need to absorb and digest—pun intended—for the present.

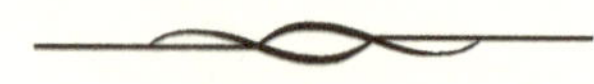

Ghrelin, leptin, and many other bodily hormones are important to wrap your mind around for sure. It is what makes the Normal Diet so *normal* in the first place! The hormonal feedback mechanisms are intricate and fascinating to say the least. Understanding that in each of us is a delicate balance is humbling and freeing.

Could the pig-out also be swings in these signaling hormones? Clearly, yes, it can and is a major cause of the unplanned pig-out.

This is what we need to know about hormones. If hormones are balanced, then all is good. If hormones are not in balance, then that is not good. Pretty easy to understand if we keep it simple.

What is less simple is how to balance these hormones and which ones are the most important. Endless books have been touting their specific rationale for a specific hormone and what to do about it. That said, I put forth here that the initial steps to hormonal balancing absolutely begins with cleaning up your diet. It makes sense to me, and I hope it does to you as well.

Out of the gate if you chase any one particular hormone, it is much like eating an exclusionary fad diet. It doesn't end good. When eating *normally*, you do not so much focus on balancing hormones, which I do agree is important, but rather returning once again to concept of common-sense nutrition and letting your body do what it does best which is—functioning autonomously without the use of physiology altering pills.

I do not feel it is too farfetched to say improvement of various nutrient intake—aka, "good diet,"—will flow *downstream* and allow for improvement of hormone upregulation in all areas involved. This is a simple truth of how we were designed to function.

Yes, our own situations and circumstances may thwart our desired outcomes, yet nobody can say that *really feeding your body well* cannot instantaneously improve your health…because it does.

Just as a fresh vegetable improves health the moment mastication begins a candy bar can instantly begin the degradation process. One improves; one hinders or hurts. Stated another way, food can be the poison or food can be the remedy. Your choice.

A real good book on the discussion of these hormones and an in-depth review of the particulars is *The Rosedale Diet* by Ron

Rosedale MD and Carol Colman. In the book, Dr. Rosedale talks about turning off your hunger switch. A solid read when you're ready for it. Of course, Dr. Rosedale has a particular hormone that he builds a case for maintaining the balance of. The book is a must read and reference tool overall. Again, when you are ready. For now, let's get back to our way, the Normal Diet.

The pig-out is no friend of ours, yet it is ingrained in our nature by and large. It will likely occur no matter what safeguards we put in place. I can say with relative authority that at some point you will find yourself at the bottom of a bowl of ice cream or holding an empty bag of your favorite goodie. Human happens!

I laugh to think that I have said on occasion, "I am going to suffer from what I am about to eat, but I don't care." Well, guess what? The near future always happens, and you will care—and suffer—and regret. Allow me to state again that mere minutes later when the gluttony of choice starts going through the gastrointestinal process, you *will* suffer. We all will and have repeatedly.

The result of the pig-out is more than feeling upset with ourselves. If that was all there was to it maybe, we could call a friend for solace and move on from that without much consequence. However, it's more than that isn't it?

Oh, the self-inflicted injustice of it all!

Yes, emotionally we can become distraught and disgusted on some level by our actions and "weakness of character." However, while that may or may not occur, I can assure you that your physiological self will need to handle what was done.

Perhaps the most common response to a pig-out is the immediate abdominal bloating and subsequent stomach pain. Belching and burping wouldn't be surprising. If a dose of sugar-laden product, then you may experience an elevated heart rate, palpitations, or heightened anxiety.

Our pig-out of choice and our general health status is always a factor in just how each one of us will needlessly suffer. Irritability, fatigue, restlessness, poor sleep, and all the rest could ensue.

Besides the acute response(s), your body may need many days to truly come back around. I find the older the person the greater and longer the negative impacts will be.

A day or so of really bad flatulence may present. Perhaps diarrhea or constipation depending. Once-quiet hemorrhoids can flair. Many experience various inflammatory issues whether it is, in fact, intestinal or joints such as hands, knees, shoulders, wrists, etc.

We are also aware that skin conditions can worsen. Psoriasis, eczema, acne, and all the rest could be triggered, and if we are to be honest, we probably knew what would happen, yet we did it and still do it to ourselves.

Without bending over backward to provide lengthy research discussions that could have you wanting to either skip the rest of this chapter or pinching yourself to stay awake, we need to simplify our thoughts on the classic pig-out. Here we go.

- The pig-out can and will happen to us all: I am not generally worried about it, and neither should you. Just do your best to make it less and less frequent. If it occurs once a month or even twice per month, that is reasonable in my book…literally.
- The pig-out can demoralize us for some time. The converse of that is the sweet "taste" of victory when you don't succumb to the pig-out and have an incredible feeling of newfound strength, confidence, and resilience.
- Feelings and emotional swings that are too far in any direction can induce a pig-out. Recognize this fact for the truth it is. Stay at "the top of the pendulum" as best able.
- Hormones will get you every time if you participate in fad or exclusionary diets. Your body *needs* all varying macro- and micronutrients. It will make you find it. The pig-out is one way to make sure you get lots of different foods the

body may need or simply just wants from embedded physiological patterns.

- Make a plan to handle the aftermath of the pig-out. That may sound odd, yet knowing that the pig-out will happen at some point, it would be wise to know how best to course correct. This may mean fasting the next day, fluids only, body movement, or otherwise. Figure yourself out and be prepared is the point.

- Get over it! So you pigged out. Go in front of a mirror. Stick your thumb in your mouth and suck on it for a while. When you are done, go make a nice salad and a batch of unsweetened iced tea or something clean and good for your body…and mind.

8

Longevity Secrets

Now, what in the world does the Normal Diet have to do with longevity? Well, besides the completely obvious benefits of living longer when you treat your body better is the simple fact that you will generally live a happier life altogether. How can I be sure? I've seen it played out over and over that's why I am so sure. When you are healthier, your brain works different. Your body works different. Your feelings and corresponding emotions are different. Your spirit is different.

Please do not take my word for it—completely change from what you are currently doing that is negatively impacting your health and life and get back to me with the answer. Try your best to prove me wrong. In many different ways, your life will be impacted for the better and much of which you can only discover as you move along.

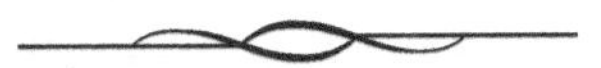

From time to time, I get the occasional cynic who is usually being followed at all times by a dark cloud who laments about "going to die anyway" viewpoint. Run from these people. If it's actually you, then run from yourself; run straight toward the new you that *you* would like to and can become. Just because you used to do or be someone doesn't mean you need to keep doing or being forevermore.

If you're ready, then change. Change your nutrition; watch how you blossom.

Now, following *The Normal Diet* gives us at the very least a shot of living long(er). It sure is not going to shorten your life! How could it? Again, the transition from what you are doing now to the Normal Diet way gives us intention, focus, healing, and ultimately, a happier healthier life, and maybe, just maybe, we learn a thing or two along the way. That's my desire, my goal, for me, you, and everyone we know and hold dear. To live very healthy and live very long.

That begs the question of, "At what point do we begin to give deep and meaningful thought to our mortality?" What would trigger such reflection? Is it at a certain age? The day your first child was born? Maybe specific ages such as thirty, forty, or fifty. Was it when you got your first gray hair or first social security check? Maybe it was the day you found yourself an empty nester.

For me, the first significant acknowledgment that we all move on from this place was when my grandmother passed away. This acknowledgment of the natural order of things morphed into painful contemplation while burying my father. Being the youngest of four boys, I have joked with them on more than one occasion that "If God plays fair, then I should be the last to go," but that's not reality, is it?

My mother told me that "When your parents are gone, that's when you start thinking, really thinking, about your own mortality. Now I'm the next to go," she said of herself.

I heard that statement through younger adult ears, and it was funny in a morbidly odd sort of way. It didn't sink in then; however, now it is. Perhaps at those time of our lives when our muscles had muscles, mortality concerns smacked us in the face in only the rarest of occasions, it is not so anymore. Those statements are more than mere words to me now.

As the years pass on, we are confronted by the stark realization that invincibility turns into introspection as we ask that timeless question "what's it all about."

While I cannot say that I have figured out the meaning of life, I have concluded that at the very least, I'll need about one hundred years of living to even grasp "it"! To that end, I am determined to, Lord willing, live well into my hundreds. I am going for it. Are you?

The desire to *live a long life* opens a lot of viewpoints, questions, "what ifs," and occasional cynicism.

"Dr. Clearie, what if you make it to one hundred but are confined to a wheelchair, have Alzheimer's, dementia, outlive everyone you know and love, etc." That's where that dark-clouded individual we spoke about earlier shows up. The anti-everything optimistic and the "sky is always falling" type of individual. By the way, they need love and mentoring as well. Some of you might be reading this, knowing I am describing you. Decide to change. It is a lot more fun this way. Yes, we will all most assuredly pass away at some point in time but live, darn it, and live well.

Truth is, I do not know how to answer these questions when they are posed in the derogatory, "what if" way. If after reading this book you find out that I suddenly keeled over as I have a history of atrial fibrillation when I was in my forties, would you be shocked? Perhaps you would smirk as you throw this material into the fireplace. I hope this doesn't come to fruition, yet anything could happen to any of us as sure as the sun shines. Life ends for each of us in turn. While clearly an honorable goal is to live as long and healthy as able, God simply may have other plans for us. Who am I to second guess the creator of *all* things?

What I do know is that you need to give your full attention to the things you can focus on *this* specific day, *this* hour, *this* moment. I hope to do the same on July 7, 2069, when I will be crossing the one-hundred-year threshold. By golly, I should already start planning because it's getting closer every single day!

Candidly, I am better equipped to address circumstances and events that are real. I cannot give energy or my time to things that are unreal and undesirable. "I can help you with reality, I can't help you with your crazy imagination" is what I like to tell my kids. They get the point.

On so many occasions, the imaginary fears, the horrible "what ifs" are only real in your mind and nowhere else. Don't give them energy. Please don't bring them to life. It is not worth it.

Given what I know at this moment, this decade of existence, I will share with certainty the desires of my heart:

First and foremost, I *do* desire to live long and live healthy. I certainly desire this for my wife, my children, my loved ones, and for you.

I desire full mental and physical capacities and a zeal for life until the very last breath. (You had better hope that the last breath I take isn't when I am adjusting you because it sure will take effort on your part to push me off your back.)

My growing belief, amidst all the advancing sickness that is currently going on around us, is that we are going to have more individuals achieve the one-hundred-year threshold. It is a growing renaissance of sorts. I am not the only one who sees such lofty attainments.

I envision, albeit this may sound like a fantasy to many, that those that do will not be on any prescription medicine at all. In fact, *that* may very well be the only common denominator between them all.

I perceive that the uber-healthy centurion bodies will be running "autonomously," meaning without outside intervention, specifically the laundry list of medicinal used today. The medicines we use today will be "extinct" at some point in the future. Those companies may even be making things like wristbands, T-shirts, the next-generation Cabbage Patch Kids or Pet Rock.

Reaching one-hundred-plus years demands a lifestyle that will allow for such a lofty goal. Don't be afraid to stick your neck out and tell others, if that's your wish, that you are going to be around a long, long time.

Here is the funny thing. The one-hundred-year lifestyle is not about avoiding the "things" that are supposed to be detrimental. What fun is in that? Of course, we all know that excess of anything, combined with not enough of the correct things is a recipe that "is hard to swallow" down the road. The gist of it all appears to be to enjoy all of God's blessings with moderation and discernment.

Many moons ago, I saw a comedian on a cable TV show talking about how people are suing Oscar Meyer Wiener because the public wasn't told that hot dogs are cancer causing and/or bad for our health. Everyone had a few laughs of course because isn't that the definition of a hot dog? Tons of instant pleasure and momentary taste bud gratification but not much in the health department. The only benefit is to the makers of Tums who will sell more product and make more money 'cause Tums is what you'll need to settle your stomach later and maybe some Imodium.

Now, this comedian lamented in much the same way as only comedians can. He went on to say that everyone inherently knows they are bad and likened these individuals to those that smoke and took issue with no warning labels. Truth is we don't need warning labels on the things that are obviously bad for our health, do we? As a boy, I knew smoking was bad. I tried it, along with Copenhagen chewing tobacco and threw up many times. Admittingly, others have not been as fortunate as I to have experienced that type of horrific and deterring event and are addicted.

The comedian concluded that from now on, to get real enjoyment, he was going to put cigarettes *in* his hot dogs, and he didn't want anybody bothering him. It is his right and is absolutely hysterical in jest. However, we need to come back to reality, don't we? Well, I have a God-given right to live as long and healthy as I can and I plan on doing it if God should so choose to allow me to be blessed in that way. If not, I am okay with it. I simply just believe that living a long healthy life and doing my part is a goal worthy of failure.

Again, I am not quite sure it's about being a non-hot-dog-consuming vegetarian and avoiding cigarettes however obvious and prudent this would be. I suspect that even considering a hundred-year lifestyle goal one would have to adapt a "flexitarian" lifestyle, which is the inclusion of varying and wholesome nutrient rich food in its as close to natural and unadulterated state as possible. This, of course, is again the essence of the Normal Diet. In addition, I suppose as you feel healthier, or to allow for further health to keep developing, one would have to be *flexible* with what they specifically need to do or not do as they discover themselves along the way.

Seemingly blaspheming is my stance that the one-hundred-year lifestyle isn't about exercising daily either. Albeit I won't leave this one to chance as consistent exercise promotes longevity as sure as consistent smoking will end it. That's not for debate. So another step in seeking longevity would be to consider a lifestyle that includes *consistent exercise and/or healthy bodily movement* throughout all one-hundred-plus years. Yes, the initial crawling turned into walking then skipping then running, which might turn into hiking and later years back to walking, which may turn into hobbling. Just be consistently exercising modestly, and we'll be promoting health with a reasonable degree of certainty. That's all I ask.

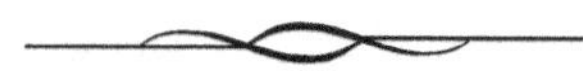

Routine chiropractic care is not for debate either. Regular chiropractic adjusting to your spine specifically and supporting structures generally enhances and maintains mobility.

But that's not all.

When you remove these restrictions in the spine, you allow for less interference, pressure, pinching, compression, chaffing, and irritation—if you will—of sensitive nerves and nerve fibers that course *through and to* every nook and cranny of your being.

At the core of living fully alive and autonomously is having free-flowing life energy and nerve impulses, traversing unimpeded from the *generation station*—your brain—down along the spinal cord and out through all peripheral nerves to every gland, organ, and tissue and then back again.

That is vital—I repeat, *vital*—to optimum function. In seeking healthy longevity, getting adjusted consistently needs to be taken seriously. Clearly the structural and biomechanical application of maintaining all moveable joints in the body is paramount, yet it bears hammering home the notion that its dramatically more important to keep the *life force* flowing freely. If the nerve impulses that control the function of your liver, lungs, or pancreas are reduced how is that organ supposed to facilitate your optimal health? Simple thinking. Tremendous health gain.

While I do perceive that all these are important aspects of living long and healthy, there are more for sure. One that comes to mind is meditation. On a broader sense another is a hobby, a passion, a reason to thrive. Your reason.

Admittedly, for years, I enjoyed the brief times in the morning when I was able to catch early morning *Today Show* news where Willard Scott gave his Smucker's brand endorsed, birthday shout-out to the centurions. Some were 101, 102, or even older. On one occasion, he had one-hundred-year-old twin men! I hadn't seen that before.

Of course, I enjoyed, and I am encouraged when he had both the husband and wife. And we all know the woman isn't really telling her true age at that!

If you have ever heard Mr. Scott, then you already know he generally had given their stated reason for such longevity which was my favorite part! One gentleman stated that it was his love of meat! Oh, the horror. One woman stated it was her daily glass of wine.

Others that filled me with gladness are those that put their faith as the paramount reason and still others spoke of deep meaningful relationship and loved ones that keep them going. Others have related an enjoyment for their life's work and still others had yet to "retire."

Ah, the purpose of life is to have a life of purpose.

To this end, I would humbly request that each of you speak health, wellness, and longevity into your lives and those you care about. Speak freely about your desire for a long and healthy life and make it so. As an experiment, go out of your way in the near future and tell another person how healthy they look. You would be amazed at how this seemingly insignificant act can upregulate the health of someone. It's not science per se; it's even more valid.

Speaking health toward someone isn't this placebo concept—it's an exchange from you to them that makes deposits into their present and future selves. Everyone benefits from uplifting another. Health improvement techniques cover many facets. Let's not be so rigid to think it's all about food intake.

Clearly, your longevity starts with the desire to be here. That's the flame that must be stoked. Becoming ambitious in this regard is first and foremost required. If you must ask yourself, "Why would I want to live that long?" then you are not thinking straight at the moment.

My conviction is that the greatest expression of gratitude and thankfulness to our creator is to, well, live long! That's what I intend to do. So should you.

9

Afternoon Basic Training

believe that *whole food, real food, God-made-food* type nutrition is the foundation upon which to maintain, rebuild, and restore our beautiful human body. Oftentimes, we find that our desire to do so and the real-world ability to do so on a consistent basis are at odds with each other. I find the afternoon lunchtime to be perhaps the most challenging aspect for many to "eat sensibly" yet is perhaps the most important consumption of the day.

How many times have you been intentional about eating well and found yourself at a midday meeting, traveling, vacation, or even just running around town when suddenly you realize "you're starving." It has happened to me on many occasions. It still does.

In the beginning, when these times occur, you may actually skip eating lunch altogether because you just don't want to eat garbage. That really is okay from time to time when you have resolve, yet you cannot routinely allow that to occur. If in a chronic and prolonged hunger mode, you will eventually cave in and run to McDonald's or any other fast food in sight. Not to mention that metabolically this may not be sustainable long term as we are not robots; our bodies require fuel. When you do go off the rails, afterward you will feel lousy in your gut and guilty in the mind. I have done it and so have you. Don't beat yourself up. Let's form a game plan here.

The typical American diet is not a good approach to adopt if you desire to maintain balance, vigor, and vitality. The American diet should be called "the perpetual holiday diet." The holiday diet is the way we *transiently* eat and drink when the holidays come around. That period of time from around thanksgiving until the new year when we tend to introduce things into our diet that we normally do not consume, think eggnog here as an example. We willingly wolf down things we normally do not eat, think homemade cakes, pies, pastries, cookies. This way of eating is not sustainable should you desire to stay healthy.

As during the holidays, special occasions such as birthdays, anniversaries, graduations, and other fun events of life will of course occur, and we should be able to enjoy the various goodies that go along with it. However, it's not only the case of *what* we eat and drink; it's how much we eat and drink during these times that takes us off course. It's the excessive appetizers that should be the meal in and of itself, the humungous plate of ham and accoutrements, the desserts and cordials and then the reheat of leftovers later that really send us over the top.

There are many other times when our diet goes south such as Super Bowl Sunday. Another diet deal breaker can be when a vacation is taken. When the children were young, we enjoyed camping. One particular area we gravitate to yearly is the South Carolina coast where we can relax as much as we want to or busy ourselves as much as we want to. It's all there for us, especially the food!

As was customary, we would pack our protein powder, our green food powder, our individual supplements. We would pack our exercise clothes. At the outset, we always planned to maintain our regular routine of food and beverage consumption. However, without checks and balances on each other, it wasn't surprising that things went sideways fast. Can you relate to this?

Nowadays, my wife and I have an agreement. When one of us starts heading down the wrong path, the other will say, "You really don't want to do that. You won't feel well later." Usually this keeps us from going crazy or as crazy. Sometimes we both get a little nuts. Afterward, we typically will feel ill, tired, just plain sick. It's the inevitable consequences of our actions. The pain teaches us so much more than words in a book ever can.

Other times that your planned dietary intake will waiver is usually, meetings, conferences, play dates for the kids, and countless others. However, these may be just singular events or one to two days max. These are okay if you are staying on the path generally.

The *path* for lunch should be *sensible*. Yes, that sounds like a large net thrown; however, when you use common sense, we end up eating *sensibly* the majority of the time. This allows for the occasional guilt-free variation in our food consumption during a holiday, vacation, and party times, etc. Does that sound like double talk? I hope not I simply want you to get the point that down deep we all know what we should or shouldn't be eating and how much we should or shouldn't be eating the majority of the time. Am I right?

Allow me to reiterate that lunchtime should be sensible, reasonable, generally good for you when walking out those wonderful ordinary days of your lives. Going off the rails for lunch day in and out rarely ends well. Staying steady for lunchtime on a consistent basis is a health game changer. Furthermore, I don't believe afternoon consumption of food needs to be a huge amount it simply needs to feed you well.

Clearly, different people have different caloric requirements to feel satisfied and promote well-being. That said, while calorie counting could add value and awareness, over time you will innately know what you need…and don't need.

Yes, lunchtime food intake should perhaps lend itself to more salad greens and simply prepared vegetables such as cucumbers, carrots, tomatoes, peppers, onions, mushrooms, and the like from my perspective. Smothering with blue cheese is my go-to when I really want to screw up a good thing! I am joking here but usually most of us add literally the worst dressings, don't we? Completely ruining the whole reason we are doing what we are doing here! Laughable… and painful…because its true more than it isn't. So watch that aspect.

Do we need to eat salads every day at lunch for the rest of our lives? Of course not, just eat daily greens as long as you would like to remain healthy! Yes, another joke here, yet the truth of it is the more green stuff we eat on a daily basis, the healthier we will be.

You rightfully should have a salad mix daily. It is really a good idea to do so! If not daily, would you consider three days per week maybe? Two? If you have less salad, you need to increase something else and that something else should be vegetables in some capacity. I am trying to drive home the green theme all through this material here. Is it getting old? Well, I am going to keep going anyway.

The point is simply to start where you are able. This is called *The Normal Diet* for a reason. Let's get me, you, us to a point where more than not we are having a clean type of lunch…and salad is a clean choice. If you feel the need to have a little chicken on it, legumes, grape leaves, then do so. Simply be clean, satisfied, and not overeating.

If not salad, then what?

Well, God made a lot of different food for us to choose from. Vegetables need to be in the mix here: asparagus, bamboo shoots, squash, string beans, radishes—I mean what's your pleasure? Pickles, sweet potatoes, celery, berries. How about avocado? Melons, papaya, raw nuts. Simply choose food made by God as much as able. We live in the real world, and at times, you have to make choices, and if you need some really good nutrition with a little "fake" food, I completely understand.

As a kinda poor example, I will share that just today my lunch was nowhere close to a salad nor enough to eat. My lunch consisted of an orange, two handfuls of raw nuts, and a "fake" protein store-bought protein-type shake. Are you horrified? Well, this book is called *The Normal Diet*, not the absolute perfect diet.

I could have, should have consumed more yet the day prior was a social gathering of the family, and quite frankly, I need to take a break from food right now ala the "pig-out" of chapter 7. I simply had too much to eat yesterday. So today, I want to allow the aftermath to recede. I had a clean shake this morning and a cup of plain herbal tea. I needed a time-out today. Tonight will be simple and clean as well. In fact, I may keep it minimal, simple, basic tomorrow as well to get myself back on track.

I even took it easy on exercising. I stretched for five minutes, performed fifteen minutes of light free weights, and did some gentle "shadow drills," which is a modified wrestling stance exercise that for me is challenging and fun at the same time.

So every day will not be perfect, yet I am asking and advising you that a good approach is to genuinely desire clean(er) real food as a majority of your sustenance. By the way, as revealed prior, it's okay to be a little hungry occasionally. Not super starving. Right now, I can feel that I could use a little something more, yet I want to give my gastrointestinal system a break. So I am drinking lemon water and enjoying life.

Do a few scrambled eggs at lunch fit the scenario that could provide nutrient, keep blood glucose levels lower and satisfy? Yes, of course. Some would argue, as I have also said prior, about allergies to certain food groups and eggs could be one of them. I understand that, yet here I am addressing those that are in perhaps free fall or in early stages of transition and have skipped meals and have a major headache. Been there? I have, and it isn't fun. So those that are doing their best to figure this whole diet thing out having eggs, even if was simply four scrambled for lunch would perhaps be wiser then fries and a Coke and candy bar. Understand?

If not eggs how about a quick piece of fish to your liking? Grass-fed beef? Oven-roasted turkey, whether warm or cold is also a simple addition that fits our plan. How about sauteed vegetables that's a great quick choice. There are many easily prepared nutrient-dense food to eat all around us, yet we go for the heart-attack foods more often than not. I am simply asking you to gently change this for lunch. You will thank yourself later.

When you start your day with clean nutrients as described in AM basic training and roll into a lunchtime salad, etc., and you do it consistently, your body will begin to respond well. You may notice yourself getting leaner in mere weeks, of course, but that's not what I am speaking to. You may have greater mental clarity. More energy. Sleep better. Have greater intimacy on all levels. Eating and drinking well actually touches upon and impacts every area of life as a human being. Prove me wrong!

I have known many to complain that they feel their intestines "clog" or become sluggish. This will usually occur because you haven't been consistent in the whole fibrous food and clean beverage concept. Modify as we have described here in afternoon basic training, and I can virtually guarantee that you will have consistent bowel movements that feel as though you have completely voided and done so easily. No pushing, suffering, nor creating future hemorrhoids and/or rectal fistulas. The output will be green as you have been eating green. You will have a sense of satisfaction in a way that's a challenge to describe. What a great conversation, right!

This is an adult topic that affects all of us so before we end (yes, another pun intended), let's press on a little here. Voiding is serious business for the body. Please take it as such. Plan for the daily ritual; do not put it off. How do you plan something like this? Just like everything else. You obtain knowledge of how your body works. If you have been living in your body for a while, then you know how it works already. For example, you may already know that coffee moves your bowels quickly thereafter, that vegetables are essential, fiber needs to be consumed, water intake is required often. You may also be keenly aware that if you are not in the privacy of your own home you cannot have a normal or complete bowel movement.

Whatever the "terms" are for you to have normal bowel movements, acknowledge them fully. If you know that corn and bread products slow down your transit time, then steer clear more often than not. If you are sure that noodles and spaghetti bloat you for days, then why suffer?

Let me state in no uncertain terms that a sensible lunch is a centerpiece of living healthy!

For lunch, you may have previously grabbed "something quick" from the hot rack at a convenience store. Maybe you threw down a couple slices of pizza, which frankly hits the spot from time to time. However, these random terroristic food attacks on yourself have got to stop!

I feel the need to repeat that if by and large you are pretty sensible day in and day out than have a meal or even a full day that is not exactly made up of the best decisions as far as diet goes you will not really feel the effects.

However, should you be one who partakes of "the perpetual holiday diet," aka the typical American diet, and *then* add the burden of an even worse splurge, it should come as no surprise that dis-ease and disease awaits. Do better. That's all that is asked of you.

10

Project Management

For a moment, let's consider you are on the outside looking in at a close friend and their current life circumstance and situation. Your dear friend has an honest-to-goodness, *sincere* desire to make changes that will improve every aspect of her/his life. They come to you and lament. They lay all the cards on the table—pour out their heart to you.

This individual asks you for help, counsel, and perhaps mentorship. A little surprised, you wonder how you could assist them when you have your own *stuff* you are dealing with. They then ask if you would be their accountability partner and could send you their daily food diary for a while.

Perhaps they want to talk once or twice a week. Maybe send you pictures of their sensible meals. Again…accountability.

Essentially, they are asking you to be their wing man. Suddenly, you find yourself as having a project to manage and your friend is that project!

In much the same way, I am asking you to be a project manager over yourself. A dear friend unto self, of course, yet also a "professional" of sorts who is determined to perform their "job" and do it well. Yes, it is a good decision to partner with someone who cares and that you can trust, but understand at some point, it's your personal desire, your own resolve that gets stuff done. You are the project manager…and the project.

The nuts and bolts of the Normal Diet is truly anticlimactic to implement. It is perhaps more effort to do what you are doing now. Said another way, the majority of people are going out of their way to make themselves feel awful. The real issue is that we get in our own way. Perhaps I should say our emotional self does and without warning we are off the path we so want to travel.

That's where the non-emotional yet highly logical *project manager* needs to step in and run the "site" accordingly.

Looking at this *business like* you can clearly see that the desired outcome is to build a healthy body. It is more than that of course because we want it all better—body, mind, spirit. For the moment, let's keep it simple. If a healthy body is our goal, then from a project management view, what are the actionable steps?

You are perhaps thinking there are many, and candidly, there may be in your particular situation. If you try and handle everything you need to all at once you would be making a major mistake. You do not need to address everything. As far as I can see all you need to really do is three things…and do them consistently.

Would you like to know what they are?

I'll tell you, but before I do, what do *you* think your top three actionable steps are? Maybe you're thinking big view like join a gym, quit my job, and take hormonal injections. Well, that's not the three I am thinking for anyone.

No, the three things every single one of us need to start on isn't exercise, supplements, and/or relationships. It's simply, get ready…

Appropriate breakfast, lunch, and dinner.

Easy peasy—three things you need to focus on, not fifty.

I'll say it again so we understand each other; the three items you need to manage right now are *nurturing* breakfast, *sensible* lunch, and *intentional* dinner.

At this moment, you do not need weights. You do not need Zumba, to jog, elliptical training, or hot yoga. All you need to do as the project manager is see to it that proper implementation of what we discuss is managed and managed well.

Recall our *commitment, congruency, consistency* discussion?

When you efficiently handle the *management* of breakfast, lunch, dinner easily within the framework of our discussions together then maybe, just maybe, when your *review* comes around you can get the "nod" to oversee the next item(s) that need to be handled. But why would you if you stink at managing these essential three?

Once these three are handled appropriately, then and only then are you ready for a promotion. Now, of course, I am embellishing a bit, however, the Normal Diet isn't called the normal cardio, the normal stretch. No, as I have said before, it is called the Normal Diet.

What crosses your lips is our focus at the moment and is paramount to achieving your health goals and desires.

If you are thinking, "I'll eat this chocolate bar tonight and run five miles tomorrow, then please think again. Not to say that wouldn't be beneficial I am simply trying to clear up any misconception that your health improvement plan at this juncture has to include anything else but food handling. The project will come to completion one day and in order to realize it, yes, we need to manage all various aspects...just not right now. The start of this project must be unequivocally consumption of food, not how many stairs you have climbed today.

What railroads many good intentions is simply taking on too much. You will not be successful if you jump to the end of the process. You have done this before. If you haven't, then you wouldn't be reading this book right now, would you? I bet one of the first things you did when getting this material was to scan for the diet menu. I've covered this a little earlier; it doesn't exist or, should I say, not the way any of us want.

Please refrain from the human primate desire to have it all in a moment's time. Accept this and you will have a sense of *calm* as you commence. Understanding this simple fact will allow this wonderful innate feeling of freedom. I share this with you as a wholistic doctor and as a human being doing my darndest to move beyond my own caveman-like tendencies.

"I want it now" was an inherent part of who we were as children. Throwing temper tantrums may have worked back then, but now, it will only frustrate your efforts.

Our feelings will always be our feelings. Our ability to better manage, handle, and cope with them, and ensuing emotions is a goal worth striving toward. The adult mind is in or should be in an ever-advancing state of maturity that it is able to logically handle the emotional surge of "now."

The now factor has ruined many good game plans of life generally. The now factor can ruin your good health as well. Instead of thinking, "*I want it all right now*," consider pondering how you will better manage *now* that will yield benefit later on today or tomorrow…which will magically turn into a "now" very soon!

Yes, you can project into a week, month, year, and even decade from now and see yourself so happy, healthy, and content with all the really good decisions you make henceforth! For the moment as we begin the process, let's allow time to pass as it should. Stay in the present and the near future, as in, a couple hours from now. Plan to feel better in three hours from now. What would you need to do, not do, to realize this?

Would a huge pasta dish washed down with cola help you in an hour from now? Of course not. Get the point?

A day last week, I was feeling considerable fatigue after seeing patients. My drive home and subsequent crawl into my home and into my easy chair was met with questions from my wife. "You look tired," she said. "Are you okay?"

I don't want to look tired. I don't want to feel tired. Do you? The simple truth is, I *was* tired…fulfilled and grateful for a purpose-filled day…yet still fatigued a bit. I gather you can attribute that to a combination of things such as the pace, pressures of the day. You could also consider I am not in my thirties anymore…or forties for that matter. However, in this instance, it was "all that" plus depriving my body of the key sustenance/nutrients it needed to perform at a high level and still have something left over for evening home life.

Is the game plan to muddle through our day to make it to the couch and then repeat and hope for the best? Is that living an abundant life? No, it is not.

On this day, I fasted through breakfast and had a lighter lunch. Of course, I was going to run out of energy, yet I did it anyway. This isn't rocket science here! Extra sleep, while I may need it from time to time, wasn't going to fix this issue. Neither would supplements. Exercise wouldn't be advised neither at the moment. I needed sustenance. I was borderline "hangry"!

I expressed to my wife I needed food *and* a foot rub. The later never came to fruition but the former did. What I wolfed down was clean, green, and nutrient-dense. It was extremely *intentional* and satisfying. Not only did that meal help me in mere minutes, it would determine how I felt in an hour or so later as the nutrients were absorbed and digested, right? In fact, it would also have an impact on my sleep, bodily regeneration, and how I performed that next morning. Is this easy to understand? I hope it is. Diet isn't something; it is everything.

My usual cutoff to eat altogether is typically 8:00 PM or a little thereafter Monday through Thursday. So that evening meal would have to, and did, provide until I got my AM intake into me some ten hours later.

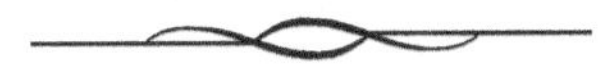

Sometimes the "project" doesn't go as smoothly as planned even when good project management is taking place. Our human bodies can be fickle. Despite all the good we do, things go off course. Conversely, all the burden we put our bodies through it generally handles it. That should surprise us yet we take it for granted…until we don't.

Even when we do, in fact, do everything correctly or as close to the bullseye as we can ailments happen. Sometimes really bad such as cancer. It's upsetting, and simply put, we do not have all the answers. What I do believe is that there is a joy and calmness that indwells when we are doing the best we can. Eating better is a large part of all that.

Gently nurturing yourself is key here.

Circling back to the pig-out discussion, I know that no sooner will someone be reading this that they…maybe you…maybe me… will be stuffing french fries in their mouth. Make the decision now that when it does occur, and it will, that you will immediately not regret nor feel guilty. Make a decision now that when that situation occurs you will forgive yourself before it hits the stomach acids.

When you feel awful from that bowl of ice cream, don't make a promise that you will never do that again because *you will* so just handle the situation with a gentle course correction. What's that correction? Well, maybe it is to *fast* a little from food. Maybe a cup of tea. It sure isn't doubling down and squeezing warm fudge from the bottle into your mouth!

All I am asking here is for you to manage the project. A lot happens during the duration of life…the project…so see to it that you manage the three most important aspects to the Normal Diet as best you are able: nurturing breakfast, sensible lunch, intentional dinner.

Let's now discuss that intentional dinner approach, shall we?

11

PM Basic Training

Where do we start?

What to eat later at night creates a conundrum from time to time. What we want to eat and what we *do* actually eat and drink collide depending on many factors; the night at hand is a major variable, what we ate prior is another, so is where we find ourselves…and who is watching…are but a few considerations.

Tell me the truth: how often do you walk in your home in the evening and before you know it you are in the pantry, fridge, and/or cooler mindlessly engulfing something you shouldn't. It's almost as if you are on "intake autopilot," and it ain't a good thing.

For the moment, let's discuss a *typical night* not the exception. Allow if you will the scenario of "Work is over, I am going home" type night that is generally a Monday, Tuesday, or Wednesday evening. In general, these should be the easiest nights to eat clean, abundantly and feel nourished. Now that is always our plan by and large yet even as you are thinking that subconsciously the "other self" cannot wait to dive into a bag of red-hot tortilla chips as you figure out what is for din-din.

If mindless predinner consumption becomes habit, it will be a challenge to change, alas, alter this habit, you must! Should your pattern become nibbling before the time dinner is ready, you are already *grained up* and kinda full and kinda feeling a tad unwell. Maybe it isn't tortilla chips; perhaps it's an ice-cold soda or beer. Could the pantry reveal an unforeseen sugar delight suddenly? Yes, it happens, and it happens often.

We can agree that one solid approach would be to take a few minutes each Sunday and decide ahead of time what you will be consuming the evening of Monday through Wednesday. That makes sense, doesn't it? In the beginning, it might feel burdensome, yet it takes mere minutes. In reality, it is just not that difficult.

The truth of the matter is that many do not stray far from repeat food groups. Yes, some are amazing cooks and create such fantastic meals, yet on average, basic stuff is consumed the first three days of each week. This has proven itself to me person after person with rare exception.

If we look at a typical *Normal Diet*-approved Monday, for example, you hopefully had a clean weekend and started Monday AM with a nice tall glass of lemon water while you are making tea or even coffee, which is perhaps more common. As that's going on you easily create a deliciously simple yet nutrient-dense smoothie.

As you get into the middle of your day, both figuratively and literally, we address the needs of our physiological selves with a greenish based ensemble as discussed earlier. Should you skip your sensible nutrient intake over lunch, it is setting you up for hormonal-induced frenzy free for all later. Yes, you can muddle through, yet I am telling you never leave your nutrition to chance or *self-imposed will* anymore. If you do, raging hormones will intercede! We discussed this a little earlier, yet it is worth repeating that seeking out a proper lunch whether it is field greens, beets, mushrooms, onions, avocados, artichoke hearts, fruits, shoots, beans, and/or whatever else floats your boat, repeated often sets the tone for the evening.

I reviewed this a little again here because if you roll into your evening with low blood sugar, your cravings will be at an all-time high and, again, your resolve low. When you walk in the door at night, you simply do not want to be "starving." Being a little hungry depending on your schedule is, of course, going to occur with some frequency in your life. Come to grips that it's okay to not be stuffed at all times.

So dinner, as far as the Normal Diet is concerned, should be absolutely, positively, *intentional*; otherwise, you will keep repeating the cycle of eating haphazardly and suffering for it. I know this to be true as a hungry version of us rarely makes the right decision. Leave as little to chance as you can. Come up with the game plan and stick to the game plan!

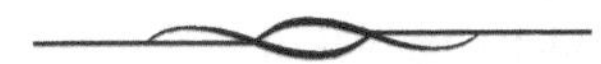

We need to be clear here in that you truly need to consume protein, fats, and fibrous carbs—all three at dinnertime. In fact, each meal should contain all three. The difference with dinner is that it lends itself to perhaps leaning more of a protein-type meal. Not always, yet it's normal that this is the case, and that's fine—really, it is. I encourage it.

A solid piece of fowl, meat, fish, or whatever is your pleasure please go have it and enjoy!

I get it some individuals are vegetarian or a version of vegetarian, and that's fine. For our talk, the Normal Diet is generally the omnivore type of people, the *flexitarian* if you will, which to say is both meat-loving and plant-loving eaters. We eat it all and eat abundantly!

The key to PM nutrition is not to over- or undereat. That's tricky business, isn't it?

If you eat the predinner snacks, you simply will not eat your meal entirely. If you do force down all of it, then it is likely you will feel bloated withing five to ten minutes of finishing. Holding your tummy as you clean and load the dishwasher just ain't no fun.

If you snack prior and do not consume all that is on your plate, you *will* be back at the freezer-fridge-pantry at some point later. You know it and so do I as history repeats itself. What is annoying is that these patterns, these habits, burn into our wiring in a such a way that these ingrained neurological pathways take over and are honestly a challenge to retool until, like a high-performing athlete, you have *trained* your brain for its "new normal."

I've stated prior that with this new way of eating, it is not uncommon to transiently have your intestines "clog" or become sluggish. You may think you must be doing something wrong. You're probably not…now; however, you *were* doing a world of hurt all the years prior. You didn't get this way overnight, and now your body must go through whatever it needs to go through. Trust me, you will be happier on the other side.

It will take time yet really focus and become aware of how your body responds to different foods as we touched on earlier.

Circling back once more to the bowel movement discussion—while consistent healthy voiding is a worthy goal to strive for and achieve, observe this bodily activity as a bellwether. The broader issue here is that regular voiding or not is a sign of whether your diet is, by and large, in the zone or not. Of course, this isn't always the case yet again it is in the majority of cases, and that's what we are discussing here.

Simply come to grips that PM eating is crucial for what transpires "later." Take to heart what I am saying here in that you will reap the reward of your intentional PM dinner habit.

I have had the opportunity to help a lot of people over the years. Not only patients who entrust me with their care but also other doctors who are searching for the holy grail of health just like the rest of us. Know that every person has an area that they desire to improve, work on, and change. Diet is virtually always at the head of the list. If this is so, why do we keep struggling and coming back to the same old issues? I wish I had a clear answer. It is different for each of us.

You may say, "My parents did this to me," or "It's the stress that makes me eat," or "I just can't help myself"; still, others say I didn't know better. The truth is that most of us do know better. All we have to do is ask our bodies. Just recently, my wife prepared a different type of dinner. It was absolutely fantastic and consisted of spices that I have not had in some time.

My wife shocked me when she said, "Let me know how you feel after you eat this." Was she joking with me? No, she really wanted to know if I felt good from this meal or if I felt disgusting. It was a rice-based meal with cooked-down greens. Yes, diced chicken was somewhere in the mix, yet also were spices, undistinguishable "granules" and other bits unknown to me yet held the promise of being uber beneficial. It truly did look every bit the part of something that was nourishing to the human body, and by golly it was! And I "felt" energized by that meal. I knew it was going to be good by the way my dogs were looking at me in anticipation!

But look, we all know this isn't always the case. We throw things down the hatch, and we suffer for it. For whatever reason, we soon "forget," and we find ourselves in the cycle, which becomes a habit burned into the part of the brain called the basal ganglia, which needs to be altered and new habits forged.

For the next week or so, simply ask yourself how you feel after each PM dinner for a while. Don't lie to yourself, just observe *self*. After you ask your body, look in the mirror and consider if what you have been eating is giving the desired physical effect you really want. After you look in the mirror, ask your loved ones if they feel you have a good dinner more often than not. Be ready for a wide variety of answers here. It isn't always what you want to hear, yet maybe it's what you *need* to hear. After these steps, why wouldn't you obtain some routine bloodwork and see what that churns up. After exhausting every earthy avenue, shouldn't you go and talk to God about it?

That's where we should have started, isn't it?

What does God say about your health, your dinners, your diet? It says in 1 Corinthians 10:31; "So whether you eat or drink, or whatever you do, do it all for the glory of God." Or consider, "The Lord will guide you continually, watering your life when you are dry and keeping you healthy, too. You will be like a well-watered garden, like an ever-flowing spring" (Isaiah 58:11).

Give that some thought each time you put something up to your lips.

Beyond that, have you ever sat quietly and just prayed and meditated on the subject of your personal health and what that means? If not, let's put down this book right now and ask God to reveal what He would like you to know about your health, food, and beverage consumption as well as anything else He would like to impress upon your heart. Do it now.

As far as PM nutrition, do your best to follow what we outlined. Also do your best not to *pregame* dinner as often while eating a clean abundant dinner with a fair blend of carbs, proteins, and fat. Feel satisfied and leave it alone. Worry not, as I bet your next meal will be here before you know it (i.e., tomorrow's smoothie or the like)!

Clearly, the PM dine situation has a significant effect and impact on your initial energy, mindset, and bodily performance when you rise that following morning. This is key so listen closely; each meal has an impact on the future "you." I mentioned prior that the future will become "now" *real soon* so eat clean in the "right now" so that your feeling amazing in the "near future now." I know how funny this sounds at the moment, yet it's a true as the sun will rise again!

Our conversation up to this point stressed the Monday through Wednesday lifestyle, and all I am asking you to do is clean up your consumption a little then a little more…then a little more. The challenge appears to be the Thursday evening through Sunday free for all that spirals us off course. Maybe not you, just everyone else…so let's talk about it.

Dinners for Thursday, Friday, Saturday can be more than a little suspect. Am I right? One Thursday night you are deep into a Sicilian pizza, and when Friday night rolls around, it's family-style buffalo wing appetizers. Saturday nights is a coin flip because *maybe, just maybe,* Friday night put your gut over the edge. For sake of argument, let's just say dinner on Saturdays are in between, perhaps part of what is on your plate is a good choice but what surrounds not so much.

Let's not forget about the alcohol choices, which if a wheat beer or grain-type spirit, it simply adds to the inflammatory response altogether.

The picture painted is truly not farfetched. You and I have lived it, I am sure, and perhaps will do so again. Why should we pretend? That would discount our life experience with the love affair for eating poorly!

In the initial stages of the Normal Diet, *clean* from Monday into Thursday afternoon has to be set in stone. Thursday evenings may be a variable. When it is simply limit the damage elsewhere. If you continue to remain unbridled, you will end up with the exact opposite of what your balanced self-desires. Tell me I am wrong. I am not…so take heed here and now.

Staying focused on PM nourishment, let's consider Sunday evening. It isn't always the case that Sundays need to be some major dining experience, yet it can be often enough. I do my best these days to blend Sunday AM to afternoon and PM food choices into a mix—match flexible situation, and I would advise you to consider the same. What this means is that I am sensitive to what the day brings forth. I may meet family or friends for a larger breakfast that my body is unaccustomed to or brunch, and if so, I reduce overall intake going into the PM timeframe or perhaps as the day develops, I might have that larger breakfast and a smoothie for lunch in preparation for a bigger dinner. I simply do not want to feel the effects of three oversized meals on a Sunday because my Mondays require high performance. I bet you can make that same claim.

Look, this discussion may seem strange to you, yet once you have the gameplan in place and stick to it, you will feel so good that you will despair when "forced" to break ranks with it all. Perhaps, in part, because you know that you just won't feel all that great on the other side of strawberry pancakes and apple fritters!

If you can remember one thing and one thing only about what type of diet you should partake of, remember that the *more you want to eat it now, the more you will suffer later*. The converse is also valid as the less you want to eat it now, the more you will benefit later.

That may sound a bit funny and more than a little bit disparaging, yet so is a diabetes diagnosis!

The Normal Diet is not taking away anything; it is outlining a path to freedom. Freedom from the odds of disease, dis-ease, and medical management beyond basic care. Here is where I need to insert the cliché that either food will be your medicine, or medicine will be your food. The choice is always yours.

You do not want colitis. You do not want multiple autoimmune flairs. You do not want fatigue, depression, anxiety, intimacy issues, or any other ailment. Not to say the Normal Diet will absolve you of all of this; I am simply saying this allows for the cards to at least be staked in your favor.

Take these odds.

To this end, *never ever* take what you consume in the PM for granted. Your body records all that is done to it for better or for worse. The playback can be amazing or simply awful. Make the changes for the love of self and the life you truly want to lead *before* you must try and save it down the road while in crisis. I say this with heartfelt love and warmth. You are so worth feeling and looking great!

12

Snacks

What's better than snacking? Not much, in my humble opinion, yet 'tis a slippery slope indeed! Let's put it in perspective. Snacking can inch us toward a multitude of undesirable outcomes such as bloating, intestinal ailments, fluid retention, aberrant emotions, reduced clarity of thinking, general malaise, and inevitably weight gain. Hence, the various need in the marketplace for trainers, treadmills, gym membership, orthopedics, meds, and all the rest.

I could keep going with the list of undesirables as *what* we snack on, *how much*, for *how long*, and each of our *individual situations* can bring us down a road we do not want to be traveling on!

I could, we all could, share scenarios wherein snacking led to downfall on the scale from "just a little off" to "it's really bad." I consulted an early-fifties athletic gentleman who had, to his surprise, gained some twenty to thirty-plus pounds over a twelve-month period or thereabouts.

How do you think he gained that much weight? Do you think he said it was from eating mutton? No. When giving deep thought on the matter he affirmed his gain snowballed from nibbling on "a little here and a little there."

Recently, a long-time patient said, "Dr. Clearie, all these years I thought the dryer was shrinking my clothes. Turns out it was the fridge…" Laughter is the best medicine, especially when it is founded on truth. Snacking leads to no good generally. I also can say that snacking is what can get to me if not intentional about nutrition consumption. In the beginning, the extra food intake doesn't seem like a big deal. The changes are almost imperceptible. A little bloating and incremental weight gain occurs kinda stealth like, doesn't it? That is until of course you "suddenly" realize your clothing doesn't fit. That usually when the self-loathing kicks in.

The fact of the matter is, most of the weight gain isn't from having six full meals per day or double dishes of meatloaf. While hands down that can do it, it is more common that mindless picking of miscellaneous food stuff is to blame. A handful of pretzels *here* and a couple of chips *there* adds up a lot quicker than one might think. So does the fake sweet tea in the cupholder of your car. Snacking late at night right before bedtime with no real rationale is also a sure-fire way to a bigger pant size down the road. Getting up and raiding the fridge for a couple scoops of ice cream during the night isn't helping neither.

In this gentleman's particular situation, we discussed desserts as being a culprit. We also discussed candies and treats in between his meals. Oh, and there was beer.

Look, America runs on snacks. The industry is enormous. Tell me how often you are told, sold, impressed upon that you should be snacking. On TV, on social media feeds, at the gas station, at rest stops, in the airports, at friends' houses, we are inundated with snack temptation.

If snacking can lead to bad things, imagine how removing these small *indiscretions* could lead to health improved. This is not some blanket statement here. If your consistent snacks are celery sticks, that's one thing. If your snacks are peanut butter cookies, well then, that's another, isn't it?

The truth of the matter is that our snacks are mostly unhealthy for us. We love them, for sure. Salivate over them, you bet! Seek them out to our own detriment. However, let's not kid ourselves; while we *want* them, we do not *need* them.

When you cut out the irrelevant snacks, you become leaner and healthier.

How would you feel, let's say six months from now, when you cut out snacking? Do you think you will be worse because of it? You may not really notice much in the beginning, but you're not in a worse health position. You are better.

How about a year without snacking? Project out five or ten years without snacking. It will have a dramatic impact, for sure. Consistency means everything. And that's why it's challenging.

I don't know about you, but what I snack on is sure to give me some version of an upset stomach in the not-too-distant future from the initial engulfment. Yes, I snack on radishes and carrots, but this isn't what I am talking about here.

I am talking about being on a drive around town or hours long trip and simply wanting something to *chomp on* and pass the time. Peanut M&Ms have been known to get past my lips on more than one occasion, and I can tell you with relative authority that after the bag was empty, my gut would hurt mere minutes later. I've proven this "scientifically" with many other snacks yet, like many the cycle, repeats itself!

Oh, the insanity of it all!

I understand that you may perhaps be waiting patiently for me to transition into a plan to thwart these snack events from happening. I am not going to pretend that anything we will discuss is ironclad because you will snack. It's human nature, I suppose.

For point of clarity, not too long ago, I was fist long into a snack albeit baked lentil chips and the thought occurred to me, "Aren't I currently writing the chapter on snacks?" I laughed to myself as I threw back another couple. So stop the guilt over it, and let's manage it to the best of our human abilities. Okay? Okay…

Our approach should be to minimize the damage as it occurs and manage the aftermath accordingly, as we discussed several times already. We could view it as a necessity to remain sane. Some recommend having one day per week that you kinda go nuts with your diet, and the next six, you get real clean. That's a great path forward, and I am behind it for sure. Can you do that forever? I can't, but I can do it for "a while."

My recommendation would be to make sure that your three meals per day are full of such nutrient density that your body does not "crave" anything. That is common sense. However, even with that, you will find something in your mouth that you will later regret consuming.

Let's take a different approach here. Consider for a moment that you are eating well for a couple weeks. Is a snack going to mess you up? No, of course it isn't, so if you're the person who is rolling along and has a snack, then it's no harm, no foul.

So let's agree that in the beginning, you simply do not snack. Just don't. Eat really clean. Eat enough so you are not hungry nor suffering and skip snacking. Surely, when you have resolve you will do it.

When you really mess up and need to "start again," then begin anew with three clean meals and no snacking. Guys, it is pretty basic stuff here, but we need to talk about it.

After you are cruising along and feeling good an occasional snack is okay, so stop beating yourself up already. The real issue is when you make every day and every "in between" snack time. Don't do that to yourself...again.

If you do snack, then get a clear zip sandwich bag and put some items in it so that when snacking happens, at least it will be thought of beforehand and hopefully better for you. You will also have a pre-determined end point.

I refer to these prepared healthy snacks as our "live alive grab bags." To feel great, you need good food. So maybe you put some sliced veggies together, and that's what's in your grab bag.

Maybe your "grab and go" is some cherry tomatoes mixed with slices of mango. Or cucumber and strawberries. Whatever is your pleasure. The point is to have health(ier) snacks planned and at the ready. Candidly, even if you do not eat what you prepared, at the very least, over time, you will be indoctrinating yourself and imbedding new healthy habit thought patterns.

What you need to keep an eye on in the beginning is spiking blood glucose levels. Our goal is to keep levels even keel over the day and not have a huge spike. So if you eat garbage snacks like chocolate candies and wash it down with soda, you're truly messing yourself up and will have to get back on the path ASAP.

Allow me to elaborate on the topic of obtaining and utilizing a glucometer. I truly feel this inexpensive device is worth its weight in gold. When I quickly and easily evaluate my blood sugars from time to time, it keeps me in check. I purchased a standard inexpensive kit from a local store, and I have had it for many years. In the very beginning, I used to check after eating, drinking, snacking, etc., simply to see how different items affected me. Nowadays, I probably check it two/three times per week.

I learned a lot about myself from doing this. One Saturday morning, when my kids were younger, I put a huge blob of ketchup on my thumb and went screaming about it to my kids, who freaked out before they realized I was joking.

I need to have some fun with this also.

But look, this is what I can tell you; the older I have become, the higher my blood sugars can go *if* I do not keep myself eating clean(er) on a day-to-day basis. Our organs are getting tired as life moves along. It is a basic fact that stuff wears out, gets burnt out, *and* I have learned that managing snacks appropriately goes a long way in maintaining balanced blood glucose levels, which clearly correlates to health and longevity. We simply cannot keep hammering our pancreas and expect it to keep up. Same with liver, kidneys, heart, etc.

Take that for how it is meant; reduce the sugar burden on your body before it is too late…and it's never too late if you can read these words.

As far as snacks go, I am telling you here and now that how you handle this area will determine how successful you are at attaining and maintaining your health goals.

I do not say this lightly.

13

A Body in Motion

No discussion of nutrition can omit touching upon exercise of the human body. They are as intertwined as anything can be. They are the proverbial *yin* and *yang*. They balance each other. And balance is what the Normal Diet is all about.

I have had many personal experiences with various forms of body movement. In earlier years, it was grueling wrestling workouts and weightlifting. This morphed into martial arts with contortions of the body that I am unlikely to perform in that manner and ferocity again.

As the years went on, running took center stage. While I have always been involved with some level of running, it was only seen as a mandatory requirement to enhance my success in other areas. I can't say I enjoyed running. It was just what I did. I might add we didn't have fancy running shoes. I recall running in high tops for many miles. I would never do that now nor do I suggest it.

Just as wrestling, weightlifting, and martial arts were a significant focus of my abilities, running, as I mentioned came to the forefront. I suddenly found myself trotting around town, through neighborhoods, along trails and toe paths. It was and still is a time of peaceful reflection.

The competitive nature with myself led me to 5K runs for fun, then another, then another. Soon that wasn't good enough, and I entered a half marathon. The feeling of conquering that milestone was enormous, but I wanted more.

In 2002, I entered and ran the Baltimore Under Armour marathon and posted a sub-four-hour time. I mention here as *I* consider this time completion as very respectable from *my* perspective. It may impress nonrunners yet not so much the elite or seasoned runners. That's okay, our competition is with ourselves, never others. It's a farce to think otherwise.

I mention my personal history with bodily movement not to show off, far from it. All looks good on paper, yet nothing to brag about. I didn't win a state wrestling title; in fact, I didn't even medal, but I did have a good run at it. It is years later with the ability of hindsight and introspection that I realize it was the "love of it all" that carried me through. Winning was the goal, I guess, yet the "grind" of it all has taught me so much more.

I did get my first-degree black belt in Sil Lum kung fu after many, many years yet have not pursued it farther. However, to this day, I carry inside me an *awareness of self* I perhaps wouldn't have discovered elsewhere.

As stated above, I did train for, enter, and complete a full marathon that brought forth a feeling of elation and accomplishment and a conquering of self that cannot be described in words, yet my daydreaming of completing a triathlon will almost assuredly stay just that.

I understand that many have accomplished much more than me or you ever will. That's okay. To be clear, exercise for our intent and purpose is not about comparing to others. We are all at different levels in this area. Different desires. Certain bodily and physical constraints that each need to consider. To this end, allow me to proceed further.

Now since that time of running a marathon my focus has now changed into, I admit, walking. Sometimes power walking, sometimes leisurely walking. Interval training with walking is something I enjoy now that I am in my early fifties. I will also share, much to my wife's chagrin, that I use Nordic walking sticks on occasion. It looks and feels odd at first but is an excellent workout for the upper and whole body. I highly recommend it.

Just a few days ago while out for a leisure walk, I crested a hill that joined with another path. At that moment, another gentleman was coming that way. As we both descended, I said, "Let's see who can walk the slowest to the bottom…" I won.

A bit of satire here, yet I want to continually drive home the point of our overall mindset with regards to every single thing we have talked about since the very first page. This is a story about you. Nobody else. Each person will do, won't do, can and/or cannot do certain things for a host of reasons. Whether food, faith, relationships, we all can do a little better or at the very least "we can do the best we can" at each stage along life's journey. Exercise is the perfect example here.

In this regard, may I suggest finding what you like to do and do it instead of doing what others recommend. I see how yoga and Pilates is beneficial and recommend it; however, it's just not for me right now. Maybe that will change.

I discuss this progression through the years from adolescent to on the fringe of an AARP membership here to show what the younger years may typically entail as it relates to exercise; that is, higher impact, intensity, stamina, youthful determination, and perhaps a streak of a competitive nature.

As the years passed, things change as nature takes its course. Just like my grandmother and my father said they would. It's not if change will come; it's when. Whether if by choice or necessity, it will come. Allow change to be a good thing in your life in this regard.

My wife and I started dating when we were both about sixteen. We have known each other for a pretty long time. She was involved in gymnastics in the early years and then onto martial arts where she exceled. However, she was never a runner and didn't want any part of it. Surprisingly, she did run with me and even committed to running a half marathon with me. One training day while getting close to our last long run of some ten miles, she tweaked her knee. Extremely painful. It was a long, hobbling walk back home. She hasn't run for long periods since. I'll admit I pushed her into doing something she just didn't like. She enjoys leisure walks, power walks, and interval walking. Now you know why I do it.

My wife also enjoys Zumba. Would she have performed Zumba years ago? I do not think so. Things change. Bodies change. As far as paybacks go, my wife pushed *me* to do more than a few Zumba classes. What's fair is fair, I suppose.

Maybe you just don't like walking, running, Zumba or yoga for that matter. That's okay. You can ride a bike. Stationary or otherwise. Elliptical machine. Aquatics, skiing, whatever. There is something out there for you to get regular and consistent body movement. That's the key…consistency.

Just this morning, a forty-something-year-old patient showed me his gym attendance statistics. In the last twelve months, he had been to the gym 601 times! That's serious commitment, and it shows.

Throughout all my years of exercise, stretching has been a component that has been a consistent endeavor. Not surprisingly, it has changed from full splits to more conservative active light stretching protocols.

Stretching is a bit more challenging these days as modest degenerative changes are creeping in. It is commonplace for us all. We can talk about this as adults and not shy away from age related reduction of bodily function.

I am not saying any of us should go "gently into the night" as much as I am being pragmatic in that our bodies change as we go through the years. That's the nitty-gritty of it all. So we had better go with it and reinvent ourselves anew as needs arise.

I was speaking with one of my older brothers some time ago. Our conversation turned to a guy we knew from high school. Let's call him Nick…because that's his name…

Nick is a little younger than my brother, yet older than me. My brother remarked that he saw this person on Facebook recently, and he looked amazing. In fact, my brother had to do a double take because this individual did not look his age at all until deeper inspection.

My brother said, "You really cannot believe how great Nick looks. He's gotta be close to fifty-eight now, and he is ripped! Looks so young. Here I am getting tired going up and down the stairs, trying to find my car keys."

Now, I have not communicated directly with this person at all really over the past forty or so years, yet I can recall at a young age this kid as an athlete many looked up to. I have seen social media postings over the years, and in them you can see him exercising, training, eating well, stretching.

He apparently adopted a healthy lifestyle and lived that lifestyle decade after decade. So it really came as no surprise that in the later stages of life, Nick is outpacing the rest of us fifty-something-year-olds. He just didn't stop.

There is something to be said about *a body in motion staying in motion.* He is consistent, and it shows. In much the same way, your consistency will show. It really will. No matter what age or health issues you have, I am telling you here and now that exercise can improve the situation.

Do you need to "be like Nick"? Well, I wish I did what Nick did all these years because I would love to look like that! So would my wife! Alas, that's not exactly the case, and hey, that's okay. Here we are now. So what are you going to do about it?

There are so many body movement possibilities these days. Again, I recommend figuring out one or two that you actually enjoy to some degree and simply begin anew and just don't stop.

Should you do something that gets your heart rate elevated? Yes, of course. Should you perspire a little. Also, a yes. Should you feel like you did something when it is completed? Of course, that's the point!

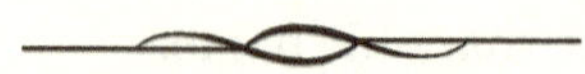

So let's begin where you can begin and put aside that someone is far ahead. You may not realize, but there are others who would like to be as healthy as you, so please remember that.

Now get moving already.

14

Desire Discipline

Our overall discussion on the Normal Diet *path* would not be complete without a straightforward discussion on *discipline*. Discipline is not something that can be purchased from Amazon.

While one could propose many aspects to fortifying discipline, such as habit formation, accountability partners, or otherwise, it truly isn't until you have a measure of innate certainty *and* set your jaw, that disciplined patterns magically present themselves. Said another way, when you have had enough, when burning *desire* comes into play, when the pain of staying the same is worse than the change, then and only then does discipline become your friend. It's true. I have seen this time and time again.

Take a moment and consider how this truth has been seen in some aspect of your life up to this point. What was the issue? How long was *said issue* a thorn in your side? Why was a particular moment or day of all days the time when suddenly you had "the burn within" to move from one place to another?

Whatever the situation may have been, can you see how suddenly and easily disciplined you became? Recognizing and understanding this can make discipline your new superpower. Entwined at the foundation of the shift is *desire*. Appropriate and well-placed desire of course is what we are referencing here. Misplaced desire can get you into bad situations.

For many, discipline can allow for a short or midterm success, but when you figure out the "why" of it all, you actually have this *innate transformation* occur in which you will find it extremely difficult, near impossible, to go back to the patterns of the person you were.

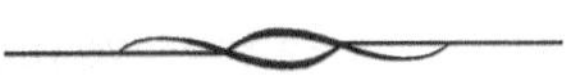

Preaching truth here, know that the mind doesn't necessarily play tricks on you. Your mind is simply trying to sort out all that is swirling around in there! So we cannot blame our minds for a shortfall in your discipline efforts! Character shortcoming usually is a target that takes blame for lack of discipline. Have you ever felt your lack of discipline in certain situations was perhaps a character flaw? Possibly a generational genetic type character flaw that has afflicted the family line for generations, now you and will negatively affect the children and children's children? Almost accepting this as your lot in life. I sure hope not because nothing could be farther from the truth!

Just this week, a woman in her late sixties on a host of prescription medications, replaced knee, replaced hip, replaced shoulder, and hurting from head to toe expressed off handily that she will take more medicine but refuses to give up all her candies, cakes, ice cream, and other treats. She blamed her grandmother and mother in a way. Clearly, she was partly joking, yet the truth of the matter is she has this ingrained belief that its true and simply the way it is going to be for her.

It doesn't need to be.

Have you ever heard that small hinges move big doors? That phrase is not lost on me, and I would ask you to meditate on the validity of that statement.

Imagine how much forward progress you would have if you somehow "found" just a little more *discipline* in one area of your life. Pick one small thing and pour discipline all over it and watch to see the momentum you gain in your life. Should you have a deep desire on top of it all, you will be amazed at your success. Together, they are an unstoppable team.

Maybe at this juncture, you might consider circling back to the commitment-congruency-consistency discussion we had prior. This all goes hand in hand.

All this said, trying to be disciplined and perfect in every area of your life is exhausting! I am not saying you cannot do it; many have, but for the other 99.999 percent of us, let's set that concept aside and chose that one thing, that one area that we once and for all decide to discipline ourselves in.

Again, the desire aspect is paramount. So much so that the area you decided on really wasn't your decision at all—it's just apparent to yourself that clearly "this" is a stain on my life that I will no longer be a party too. In fact, it's as if the decision was made for you from a higher power, and at this moment, you just simply have come to agree with what you have known for quite some time.

I hope all that doesn't seem too farfetched. It isn't yet let's bring it together in a real-world way with the topic at hand—your consumption of food.

How many people do you know make announcements everywhere they go that they have decided to, let's say, go vegan, low-carb, high-carb, no fruit, only fruit, mega fat or no fat, high protein, no protein, or any combination thereof? Tons of people, right? Self-included is what we all should be thinking right now.

And looking down the road a couple months, weeks, and perhaps mere days, we find it is typical that the *exact opposite* of the intention is actually taking place. The no-fruit proclaimer is having a huge fruit smoothie. The vegan is at a barbecue joint. The low-carb is consuming a whole loaf of bread. Its human nature and its comical.

The truth is after our proclamation, and that moment we do otherwise, by and large, we detest ourselves. Maybe not you, but this is usually the situation I have been privy, too, time and time again. It is tiring on so many levels continually going up and down this roller coaster and adrenal depleting self-loathing. So let's agree to stop the personal beratement and start simply seeing it all for what is is…we are human.

In Romans 7:15–20, it says, "I do the things I don't want to do and don't do the things I do want to do." That's a simplified version of it, yet it's the timeless truth of what being human nature is and the struggle to grow beyond it.

Facing battles on every front was perhaps the folly of my youth; now I acknowledge and work *with* that well-placed desire and appropriate discipline and I can (1) generally *flow through* life with less stress and greater joy, (2) forgive myself quickly when I fall short, and (3) regroup timely while knowing that "human is as human does."

What if you asked me if making the bed each morning would lead to a happier, healthier life? I would have to say if that makes you feel empowered and you have an inner awareness that this needs to be done, then of course in that small way, your life would improve!

Whether something big or something small any endeavor has the potential to move the needle forward. In this case, we all know there is no better feeling then to get into a well-made bed the next night! Am I right?

How about if you decided that before you tackled the reduction in your daily diet Mountain Dew intake that you needed to address and get consistent with, keeping your side of the bathroom sink clean. So be it! Who am I to tell you otherwise! Tackle what your heart is telling you to tackle—not avoiding the elephant in the room, of course, yet let's go get that first small success then the next and the next… It's empowering!

Bringing it back to dietary intake, how about laying all your cards on the table and see what you are willing to tackle? What area of consumption do you have a desire to transform, alter, retool?

Perhaps you key in on *when* you eat versus *what* you eat in the beginning. Some utilize a technique commonly referred to as *intermittent fasting*, which feels like another type of program that you will let yourself down with. So let's simply call this for what it is, more of an "eating window." Not forever, just for, let's say, this week, you decide to not consume anything after 8:00 PM and not before 7:00 AM. This is an example not exactly a suggestion, although it's a pretty good idea in my book, *and* this is my book.

Maybe you feel led to bless your food and praise God for whatever is in front of you no matter if it's a salad or buffalo wings. There is power in blessing your food and beverages; give that some thought. See *this* also as the truth it is.

Another consideration besides altering food types and beverages you ingest is choosing to recuse yourself from the *amount* consumed altogether. Perhaps you limit or reduce the size of the plate, bowl, or glass size. Imagine if you consistently left 10 percent of all food left on your dish unconsumed. Yes, I know you would be throwing out a lot more food as it would end up in the garbage yet are you a human landfill? No, you are not, so let's not worry about saving the planet at this moment; let's save yourself, then the healthy *you* can save the planet.

Are you beginning to see just how small decisions made lead to significant life-altering outcomes? We all know this as fact, yet we feel the need to push a boulder uphill as if that's something more to cheer on, then making a decision to not eat within three hours of bedtime.

While we cannot discuss every possible angle to take, I bet at this moment you already know what you simply had enough of and are chomping at the bit to do what it is that needs to be done.

Discipline is good for us. Leverage your understanding of this!

Truth is, most of us suffer many times over before we face whatever it is that we need to. Back in the summer of 2014, while on vacation, I asked myself why I was drinking alcoholic beverages. The problem wasn't the alcohol; the problem was that I knew my body and the last thing it wanted was an adult beverage.

I just didn't feel good from it. It didn't relax me. I wasn't happier necessarily either. In fact, all it did was make me tired and bloated.

Instead of playing on the beach, I slept on the beach. Instead of reading the books I was looking forward to, they remained put away. Instead of going for nighttime walks with my lovely wife, I went to bed early.

During that time, I declared to myself that I just wasn't going to drink again for at least a year. Some would say that seems like a punishment of some sort. It wasn't. What it was, was long past due. When I took a mature minute the honest-to-goodness inner dialogue with myself was that I didn't like the way I felt when drinking nor the way it kept me from living and enjoying life to the fullest. Alcohol took me away from what I truly desired. Same whether we are discussing ice cream, chocolate cookies, bagels, pizza, and everything else that has some sort of promise yet falls flat in reality. I was done with it.

So did I go a full year without adult beverage consumption? Yes. I will share that after that year I did have alcohol again. After a few months, I made a decision to just not partake. I didn't have any for about seven years.

I still went out and had great times with my wife, colleagues, and friends. I still purchased wine for my wife. Made mixed drinks for others. I just decided this wasn't for me... I joyfully became the designated driver. I was awake, sharp, content, happy, healthy, spirit-filled. Alcohol did none of that for me. Either does eating poorly.

Have I had alcohol again since? Why, yes, I have. The funny part about it all is when I do, my now-older young adult children are kinda surprised. Think about that. My kids grew up without much of that in the house and generally around their environment. What was around and still is leans toward the smoothies, tea, whole food supplements, exercise, church, structure, and all the rest. Not perfectly, mind you, yet in the forefront.

Your desire combined with discipline can clearly move mountains. When it comes together, those gray areas of your life are easily handled. Maybe not so much right at first in some cases yet it really could be that simple.

I am asking you to embrace discipline in your life. Yes, the inner child may throw a fit from time to time-keep the faith, the noise rattle will fade.

The center piece of a healthy life is maintaining a healthy diet. In doing so, you *feel* good physically, mentally, and emotionally. Gives you a leg up in handling other areas of your life requiring full attention and clear mindedness.

May I conclude here that there is absolutely no downside to appropriate discipline in your life. Only tremendous upside. Desire this.

15

Closing Arguments

As we barrel headlong to the finish line, I have no doubt that you may have areas you are unsure about, would like more input on or even disagree with some or perhaps all that we discussed. All along, it has been your right to burn this book at any time!

My ultimate desire with writing the *Normal Diet* was to provide a *foundational* understanding of how to simply eat well and thrive. Somehow, we have made nutrition so convoluted over many years that we find our country's health grave as a whole.

Perhaps this was the intent as medicine can fix everything right? Well, that approach is not working out so well, is it? I am not saying you don't need medicine. I am simply saying that perhaps you would, or may require less if you prescribe to the Normal Diet tenants. Perhaps the medicine would have less work to do if your *human being* was fortified better.

Throughout this book, my intention has been to provide a real-world discussion about nutrition—your nutrition and perhaps even more important a renewed mindset to go with it. My hope is that you would come, have come, to your own conclusion that more often than not, choosing real food over fabricated food will improve your odds of living healthier and presumably longer than you would otherwise.

I tried not so much to speak from a position of authority—rather as someone who has been where you may be at because I myself "have been there" and could be so again at any time. To this end, every word and thought pattern was chosen with great care. I pray nothing I have shared, said, discussed was taken out of context, or caused you to feel guilt, shame, or inadequacy. Life is too short for that!

I do hope what we covered fostered deep personal reflection. If you have taken stock of self, if even for the briefest of moments, then my work is done here.

I Just want to see you take good care of yourself.

The basic outline of the dietary considerations I have talked about are not *my* rules. They are more like practical guidelines that just make sense in a world that's lost view of the lighthouse long ago. In fact, truth be told, I am truly no expert on the matter of nutrition at all. Perhaps I should have said as much so in the brief synopsis affixed to the inside front cover. But how would I sell books?!

If you want to know who the real expert is on nutrition *and* a whole lot more *and* whose book you should immediately purchase if you have not already done so is…God and His book is called the *Bible*.

We would be wise to follow His leading a bit closer than perhaps we currently do. Please do not think just because my name is on this material, I am immune. I have my areas of challenge and you have yours…and God has us both, has us all, covered from start.

Far from that place of being the so-called authority, more like an *end user* myself of this overall discussion, please allow me to clear up a few things written here. Perhaps also a bit of clarification on some topics not really deeply discussed until our next publication hits the shelves.

Here we go:

- For one, I get the question of coffee day in and day out. To the point, coffee is poison. No two ways about it. You know it. I know it. Everybody knows it. Doesn't matter what any purported research claims conclude, we all know in our inner person that coffee isn't good for the human body.

- Alcohol is another toxin/poison that the vast majority partake in. It is simply foolish to drink. Alcohol does not do the body any good. No benefits whatsoever from an adult perspective. Yes, we can make light of many aspects to the societal benefits of alcohol and all the fun we have when indulging; however, at the end of the day, we are better off without it. Enough said on this.

- Yes, you may get the feeling that I view nutritional intake is in fact more important than exercise. Let me be perfectly clear because I do not want to leave anything left to the wrong interpretation when I say, in no uncertain terms, that out of the gate nutrition *is* absolutely more important than exercise. Shocked? I hope not. If it was, you would be reading a book called *The Normal Exercise*! This is one of the next books that will be released, *but* that said, for now, nutrition is and always will be preeminent! When I was training for a marathon, I actually gained over 12 lbs. I got heavier while running 10 miles per day! You tell me why...

- You won't overeat protein in your lifetime. No matter how much you think you will, you just won't. You *will* consume way too many garbage carbohydrates. Do I have to quote a research study here, or can we just agree on this one? So just eat more protein from all sources, and naturally, you will feel more satisfied altogether.

- Nowhere did we "deep dive" on fats. That was intentional for now. There are so-called good fats and bad fats. Within these two, we can further classify fats. Have we lost our minds? Look, "fats" are essential to life. The types of fats that are corporately produced are typically life shortening-type fats. The types God made are life-enhancing. I have not strayed from my natural perspective on this matter. Fats that are inherent to wild caught fatty fish enhance life. The trans-fats in our chips or that cook our fries on the other hand is another matter. Again, I suspect I will have an entire publication on this topic down the road, Lord willing.

- If the idea of going easy on consumption of food first thing in the morning feels counterintuitive, know that in some cases, you may be right. How would I know your circumstance? I will say rather than think of a reduction in quantities of food or fasting being performed, consider more of a consistent pattern of routine intake that you know works well for your body. It may take some time to get it straight, but that's okay. To have a continuous twenty-four-hour feed cycle is simply just no good no matter which way you look at it. It's the quality of food with much better nutrition is our focus.

We could go back and forth at great length with these bullet type of discussion; however, at the end of the day, at the end of the book, we need to take a moment and ask ourselves, "What am I going to choose now?" Am I going to choose to be the same person I was who did the same things I used to and suffer round and round with the same "stuff" over and over, *or* am I ready to take this opportunity to start loving and respecting myself the way I should have all along?

I know that to be so bold as to put forth a question like this borders on *none of my business*. And you would be right! But what is my business is saying it like I see fit, and then you can do what you will.

I honestly would enjoy hearing how what I have written throughout may have somehow impacted or touched your life. While I may not be able to respond to all correspondence, please know I will read each and every one and take what's said to heart.

I, for one, have learned much during the course of the writing of this material. Honestly, I needed to hear this in total as much as I felt compelled to write it. This material is as much a reflection of who I am as much as who I hope to further evolve into.

Finally, I must admit I have much more to say on the topic of natural health and wellness than what we have covered; *alas*, here is where we leave our friendly conversation for now. I hope that what we discussed has left you with a different perspective and new understanding of nutrition. It feels like I have relied on *hope* a lot in my life. Giving this deep thought, I know why. It is because *hope in the Lord* and His word is my point of reference, and with that said, my *hope* for you in my final tiding is that I pray you live the rest of your days in peace, joy, and great health!

My best to you,
Dr. Glenn A. Clearie

ACKNOWLEDGMENTS

Lacking a perfect internal recall system, you may call it memory, I have accumulated what I believe to be perhaps one of the most important aspects of this writing, that being paying homage to others who have made this book, more specifically my life, abundantly filled.

My daughter Jacqueline, my eldest, who has borne and will continue to bear the brunt of my learning the ropes as a father. I suspect this will be the case as long as I live. Each new stage for her is a new stage for me. My work on this book and my craziest of ideas have been, in large, shared with her while sitting on the corner of her bed. Her wide-eyed look of disbelief and an occasional "You can't say that" has made me fine-tune my positions and postulations on many occasions.

My daughter Olivia, whom no observation would escape her scrutiny or contemplation. From my view, your God-given gift of discernment and ever-growing wisdom continues to fascinate me. You so see the world as it could be, should be. Much of my writings could be seen as a plagiarism of one of your notions at its most basic level. You make me think—and rethink. I thank you.

My son Drew or, as we like to refer to him…Drem, his alter ego. His calm demeanor and love of the sport wrestling has taught me that "it will all shake out." Clearly, nutrition is important, but you have shown me that passion and determination is food for the soul!

My wife, Stacey, who has been there since the beginning and helped me make the Double Whopper with Cheese sandwiches at

Burger King, where we met when we were sixteen, *I thank you*, my dearest and the fairest in the land. I thank you for helping to nurture that boy into the man he is today. I owe much, if not all, to you. The writings, this book is much *our* story of evolved thinking, a step-by-step progression that has taken more than thirty years to get here.

My patients, who have been the focus of my desire to seek the truth about all things edible and nutrient-rich. Without whom, this book would be just a written conversation with myself rather than for you. I pray these ramblings of an aging chiropractor would reach more people and transform those in ways I could never have even dreamed. Many want to make a difference. Few are given the satisfaction.

I thank you all.

ABOUT THE AUTHOR

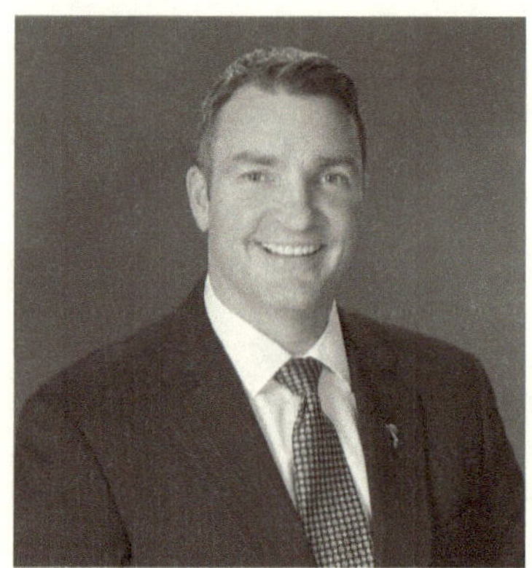

As a doctor, author, and speaker, Dr. Glenn Clearie continues to inspire others with his passion, knowledge, and common-sense approach to health, healing, and thriving. Dr. Clearie is a boots-on-the-ground clinician, practicing in the beautiful Lehigh Valley of Pennsylvania, and to date has published some seven hundred articles and counting in his Natural Perspective health column. *The Normal Diet* is the first of many anticipated publications as Dr. Clearie launches headlong into the next chapter of his highly successful professional career. Glenn, his wife Stacey, and three adult children reside in Northeast Pennsylvania.

www.ingramcontent.com/pod-product-compliance
Lightning Source LLC
Chambersburg PA
CBHW022019150726
47990CB00002B/726